Auti
Asperger's Syndrome

*The Easy-to-Understand and Practical Guide
for Parents, Educators, and Those
with Autism Spectrum Disorders*

*What if you could really
understand and connect
with autism?*

TIAGO HENRIQUES

DISCLAIMER

The information presented in this book is not intended to replace the need for a consultation with a qualified medical Doctor and should not be regarded as individual medical advice. The information presented in this book is not and should not be considered an attempt to practice medicine. The author has made every effort to ensure the accuracy of the information contained in this book and that they were accurate and correct at the time of publication. The author does not assume and disclaims any liability to any party for any loss, damage or inconvenience caused by errors or omissions in this book, whether these errors or omissions are the result of an accident, negligence or any other cause. Any references to persons or brands are merely illustrative.

COPYRIGHT NOTICE

Table of Contents

Introduction

How would your life change if you could see the world through the eyes of autism? 5

Chapter 1

Different, Strange, or Fascinating? 9

Chapter 2

How Does the Autistic Brain Work? 17

Chapter 3

The Difference Between Concrete and Abstract Thinking — The Secret to Communicating with Someone with Autism....................26

Chapter 4

Emotional Intelligence for the Autistic — yes, it's possible for someone with autism to understand emotions 34

Chapter 5

Unraveling the Mysteries of Stimming 78

Chapter 6

Sensory Hypersensitivity — A Fundamental Aspect of the Autistic Brain Frequently Ignored 84

Chapter 7

How to Identify and Stop a Meltdown?............................ 99

Chapter 8

Favorite People — Myth or Reality?............................ 110

Chapter 9

Special Needs of the Autistic and How to Meet Them.................. 119

Chapter 10

The Difficulties of Receiving an Official Diagnosis 137

Chapter 11

A New Vocabulary... 142

Chapter 12

Why Can We Have Hope for Improvement? 147

Appendix

Four supplements that relieved the symptoms of autism in published scientific studies... 154

Other Books and Projects by Tiago Henriques 167

Did You Know? 172

Bibliography 174

Introduction

How would your life change if you could see the world through the eyes of autism?

"Your child has autism." These words devastate a parent.

But what is autism?

When you look at a list of symptoms you get a general idea. But the real questions persist:

- What goes on inside my son's brain?
- What is it like to live in his world?

What if you could understand his mind?

Imagine how easy it would be:

- You would be able to **predict** nervous breakdowns and panic attacks before they occur.
- You'd know how to react.
- You **wouldn't feel helpless anymore**.

How valuable would that be?

These intense periods of distress are usually called meltdowns.

This term, meltdown, is used for two things: to describe the intensity of an autistic breakdown and to describe the fission of a nuclear reactor.

Can you spot the connection?

If you have witnessed a meltdown I'm sure you can. As a parent or educator, watching a child beating himself, screaming or even throwing things, can be as scary and confusing as witnessing the fission of a nuclear reactor. But **your life could be different.**

Imagine if you knew what to do at these times of extreme distress. You wouldn't feel helpless anymore. You would rise to the challenge and guide the child through these intense breakdowns, unharmed.

"What a relief that would be," you may think, and you're right. But, let me ask you this: Do you know anyone with this skill? Very few people have it. It's that unique. And a very important one too. Why?

Because, when you know **what to do**, and what **not to do**, during a crisis: you transform the child. He begins to feel comfortable in your presence, even during most meltdowns. This is as vital as you can imagine.

For example, many parents find it difficult to create a strong emotional connection with their autistic children.

But what if he can feel you understand him at a level no one else does?

In this case, strong mutual feelings of attachment will take root in both of you. Chapter 8, on favorite people, explores this unique kind of bond in detail.

Maybe you have been told such a connection can't be created with someone with autism. Fortunately, that's not true. Not at all.

Do you keep doubting yourself as a parent?

I'm sure you love your child and want the best for him. That's why you are reading this book. But autism, including Asperger's Syndrome, puts you in a difficult position because your child doesn't experience the world the way you do.

Many common-sense things a parent does to express his love backfire when done to an autistic child. It's as if you were using what you know about driving cars to pilot a plane. It won't work. You need a different skill set.

But what if you had those skills?

You are about to find out. Why? Because this book was built so you can acquire them fast.

For example, in chapter 4 you will understand why the autistic brain finds it so hard to comprehend emotions. At the same time, you will be learning how to explain what emotions are, and how to deal with them, in a simple and autistic friendly way.

Wait, explaining emotional intelligence in a way the autistic brain can understand? Yes. And I believe that's the first time such kind of information will be presented in writing.

You will be reading the techniques, acquiring the skills, and understanding why they work. All this from the perspective of the autistic brain.

Everyone needs to feel loved, including those on the autistic spectrum. Not just a frail love, but the kind of profound humane connection that's built upon true understanding and mutual care. Someone with autism desires this just as strongly as you do, even if he doesn't know how to express this need in his own words.

Are you an educator, a health professional or married to someone on the spectrum?

Each of the principles detailed in this book will be presented in a practical way. Anyone who interacts regularly with someone on the autistic spectrum will find these principles readily helpful and enlightening.

Are you on the spectrum?

Then prepare yourself to understand your brain in a way you may have never thought possible. Since this whole book was written in an easy-to-understand manner, you won't be bored by abstract language — the kind of language you can't readily see in your mind's eye.

Instead, we'll be using words and comparisons you can readily visualize. You will find this style of writing won't waste your precious mental energy or make you nauseous like many scholarly books do.

To all my readers,

However autism as entered your life it's my hope this information will change everything for the better, for you and your loved ones,

Tiago Henriques, Independent Researcher, Educator, and Author.

Learn more about me, my books and my work at the end of this book.

Chapter 1

Different, Strange, or Fascinating?

None of us is equal. We have different hair colors, skin tones, heights, and weights. However, certain differences *are more different* than others. Wait, what?

Think about hair color, for example. If I have black hair and you have red hair, our hair colors are *different* but none of us find this *strange*. Now, imagine that someone with blonde hair comes to meet us. Again, this color is *different* but not *strange*.

Over time we become used to all these differences, whether they are in the color of our hair, weight or height.

However, imagine one day we see someone with naturally *green* hair. Green? No doubt this is *different*, but it is a *different* different, don't you agree? It's *strange*.

But why is green hair strange? Because *nobody* has it.

The same goes for height. Someone 10 feet tall wouldn't just be *different*, he would be pretty *strange*.

Why am I mentioning this?

Because scientists are very interested in the human characteristics that escape the norm. We may call them strange, but an investigator calls them *fascinating*.

In fact, someone with green hair or 10 feet tall would be fascinating to meet. We would want to understand the reason for this person's difference and how it affects his life.

Eventually, we might even wish we could be 10 feet tall or have green hair. Suddenly the *strange* would become *desirable* to us.

What is a syndrome?

A syndrome is a set of *strange* characteristics.

These characteristics are different enough to stand out. Moreover, although they don't appear to be directly related, **they frequently occur together in the same person**.

For example, suppose a scientist named John Walks observes how most people with green hair tend to have 4 fingers on their right foot. This *is* strange.

John thinks so too. He stops and rationalizes: "I don't know why, but there seems to be a connection between green hair and feet with four toes. Maybe both are related to a common gene." John decides to look closer at this group of people.

Over time, he notices something remarkable: most of these people share a third common trait! They are all able to get their driver's license quickly, effortlessly. It seems they were born with the gift of driving vehicles. They get inside a car and they drive it like if they've spent their whole lives doing it.

Well, now things are becoming more and more fascinating. John decides to submit his research for publication in a reputable scientific journal.

A few weeks after being published, John starts getting emails from researchers around the world. To his amazement, many others have been intrigued by green-haired and four-toed people, but they had never realized there was a connection between these two traits and the ability to learn to drive quickly.

To John's surprise, doctors, scientists and other researchers worldwide are beginning to refer to this set of 3 strange traits as "Walks' Syndrome" in honor of John Walks' discovery.

Asperger's Syndrome

Hans Asperger lived between 1906 and 1980 and for two decades was in charge of pediatrics at the University of Vienna. Through his observations, he noted that some children were *different*. However, these differences were *strange*.

What differences did he observe?

For example, he noted that some children had a hard time making friends with children their age. Hans Asperger was intrigued because these children had a normal intelligence. In fact, Asperger called them "little teachers" because when he talked with them about a subject of their interest, they were able to explain it in detail.

When he examined these young boys more closely, Asperger noticed they had many difficulties in understanding non-verbal communication. It seemed that they paid attention only to what they heard, regardless of the other person's facial expressions, body language, or tone of voice. Moreover, they seemed to find it very difficult to express empathy and to be interested in others and were clumsy.

Hans Asperger wrote more than 300 scientific papers, many of which on autism, as a result of his observations. However, his research only received due recognition after his death.

Nowadays, many researchers are *fascinated* by these *strange* traits originally described by Hans. Over time, the scientific community began to say that people who had this set of characteristics had "Asperger's Syndrome," in honor of Hans Asperger's original work.

Hans was not the only one to notice this set of traits. Other researchers had also referred to them, but none of them gained the same notoriety as Hans Asperger.

But Asperger's is only one of the more moderate forms of autism.

What is autism?

As discussed in my book on safe supplementation with high doses of vitamin D and vitamin K2[1], our brain is made up of billions of cells that specialize in processing information. These cells are called neurons. If we imagine that the brain is a company[2], we can think of each member as representing a neuron. And, just as every employee in the company is assigned to a department, so every neuron in our brain belongs to a module. In what way?

For example, a large company has a marketing department, a human resources department, a customer service department and so on. Likewise, our brain has areas specialized in processing the sounds we hear, areas dedicated to determining whether these sounds originate from other humans or from another source, and areas focused in deciphering the verbal messages these sounds contain.

In addition, we have another fascinating area, the area responsible for extracting subtle messages present in the tone of voice and in the facial expressions used by other people.

For example, imagine that you approach someone you know and say: "Hello, how are you?" This person might respond with: "I'm fine. Thanks," but is he being honest? It depends.

To understand the meaning *behind* the words, you pay attention to his tone of voice and facial expressions. Has he spoken slowly, in a low volume, while frowning his face? Then you know that *he is not okay*. The result? As the good friend that you are, you will adjust your words accordingly.

Your next question will probably be: "I see you're not feeling well today, what happened?" And the person will vent and feel relieved.

---

[1]   Available   for   purchase   on   Amazon.com   trough   this   link: https://www.amazon.com/dp/B07F7LPWML

[2] A view popularized by Temple Grandin in her book *The Autistic Brain*. One of the books I recommend you read if you haven't yet.

However, had he spoken in a lively tone, with a big smile on his face and you would believe he was being truthful.

You may haven't even noticed it, but inside your brain, all this information has gone through several departments, or areas. This happened automatically. You didn't have to keep thinking about it, wasting your mental energy. You read his nonverbal cues in real-time. Why? Because you don't have autism.

An autistic brain is different. How much different? Well, the areas related to communication, socialization and emotional processing, among others, don't develop properly. Because of this, the brain of an autistic person finds it difficult to process the information present in a subtle facial expression or in a small variation in volume or tone of voice.

The Autistic Spectrum

Autism exists in a spectrum. This means a person may be more, or less, autistic.

For example, someone with a moderate form of autism — often called Asperger's syndrome — may have a hard time understanding the hidden nonverbal messages behind a simple "I'm fine, thanks."

It may take him a few minutes to compare this "I'm fine, thanks." with other similar expressions he has heard throughout his life. He needs to make a **deliberate effort** to think about the underlying meaning of the words he hears.

However, sometimes the autistic person doesn't have the time to think about it for as long as he needed and must risk a reaction. Maybe he decides the person was being honest, so he fails to ask, "What's wrong?" since he didn't detect the depressing tone of voice.

The other person, though, regards this indifference as contempt and concludes the autistic person is cold and disinterested in the affairs of others. This isn't true. What happened was simply the result of a different brain.

Back to the analogy we borrowed from Temple Grandin, it's as if a customer service department kept receiving complaints about one of their products. But no one seems to care. No spokesperson comes to the media to apologize. The company fails to react. As a result, buyers feel cheated and assume the company managers couldn't care less about their customers.

However, what is really happening? As it turns out, the customer service department isn't communicating the complaints to the direction of the company. The direction has no real notion of the seriousness of the problem.

But not all autism is like this. Some people suffer from a deeper form of autism.

They may be unable to speak or even react to external stimuli. Going back to our analogy, it's as if the customer service department didn't even exist. Any complains just pill up in the mailboxes.

Autism, however, doesn't affect just communication and social intelligence. The reason why these are its most well-known features is that they are the easiest to spot by an external observer.

What other areas are affected? For example, those related to the processing of sensory information, such as temperature perception, or the areas related to impulse control, among many others we will be investigating in the following chapters.

At the same time, areas related to the processing of musical theory, mathematics, art and design, and comprehension and production of written material, may have developed far beyond the norm.

This means that you may have someone with a more moderate form of autism, like Asperger's syndrome, who plays piano and composes music like a musical genius, but who is unable to notice whether you are using irony or being sincere.

How widespread is autism?

Currently, mild or profound, autism affects 1 in 68 people. Boys being 4 times more affected than girls.[3]

However, researchers estimate the real number may be higher. Why?

Due to the nature of moderate autism, it sometimes remains undetected. Not that the unusual traits aren't noticed, it's just that autism tends to be mistaken for other more well-known disorders. And, in many cases, it *promotes* them. How?

Someone with Asperger's may develop depression far more easily due to his difficulty in processing emotional information. Sometimes the depression is detected but not the underlying autism. As a result, the person fails to respond to the treatment.

---

[3] Article: https://www.ncbi.nlm.nih.gov/pubmedhealth/PMHT0024869/

Asperger's syndrome is often the wizard of Oz behind the curtains. It can be handled, but first, we must realize it's there.

Likewise, you may not be sure of your diagnosis or the diagnosis of your child. You notice some characteristics, but you aren't certain about others. How do you solve this problem? By abandoning this way of thinking completely.

A new way of looking at autism

In this book, instead of looking at a list of symptoms, we will be looking closely at what goes on inside the head *and body* of someone with an autistic brain.

This will allow us to understand *what to do* to deal *with each specific trait* of the autistic personality.

Why is this approach better?

For example, imagine that your child has what is called sensory hypersensitivity. This means that the areas of his brain related to the processing of one or more senses are super sensitive.

Perhaps this is the only symptom you can notice in your child, besides some minor difficulties with social interaction and a fascination with Star Trek. If this is the case, your child will never receive a diagnosis of autism. But the problem of hypersensitivity remains there, and you need to know how to act to minimize the difficulties it causes.

Furthermore, equipped with the correct knowledge about autism, you'll be able to understand the hidden message behind odd behaviors like stimming — the unusual and repetitive motions that characterize autism.

You, an autism specialist

Once you know how to handle each of the autistic traits, you will become an autism specialist.

None of the symptoms will be *strange* to you, just *fascinating*.

It doesn't matter what's the trait, or to what degree it's present. From the moment you understand what is happening, you will know how to deal with any of the traits, in anyone.

It could be you, your child, your student or a co-worker. You'll spot a behavior and you'll immediately understand how to react. With the right set of tools, it becomes that simple.

This holds true even If you are the one with the autistic traits. This book will allow you to look at your whole life from a completely new perspective.

Imagine looking back and find yourself saying, "Oh, so that's why I..." or: "now I get it! That's why I acted like this when... "

Moreover, equipped with the knowledge this book gives you, you will be able to make better decisions. Decisions that will benefit you and anyone around you with autism, especially those under your care. In a way, you'll be able to predict the future much better, knowing which behaviors will end up resulting in a meltdown and how to make better choices.

You'll also be able to separate bad advice from good advice much easier.

Chapter 2

How Does the Autistic Brain Work?

People seem more attractive in a bar. Why?
Because one of the properties of alcohol, upon entering the brain, is to disturb the area responsible for detecting asymmetry in people's faces.

We find a person more attractive if the right side of their face looks like the left side. This makes sense. If a person has the right eye larger than the left eye, we don't find her as attractive as if her eyes were the same size. The same happens with the mouth, nose and all the other details of the human face.

How is this evaluation made?

When we look at another person's face there is a specific part of our brain that answers this question:

- From 0 to 10, where 0 means "completely different" and 10 means "perfect symmetry", what is the degree of symmetry in this person's face?

If that area of the brain finds the answer to be 10, this will have a positive influence on our perception of this person's beauty. But, if the answer is 0, the influence will be very negative. How does alcohol affect this process?

If you drink too much alcohol your brain will give a perfect 10 to everyone.

But that's not the only way alcohol affects the brain.

When someone drinks too much alcohol this also influences their motor coordination, their reasoning, and their ability to inhibit reactions — their self-control. You don't expect a drunk person to be able to keep an intelligent conversation going, to walk straight or to control his urges.

This example helps us understand that our brain has many areas and that when one of these areas is affected, it completely changes our set of abilities and personality.

How does this relate to autism?

In chapter 1, we briefly reviewed how the areas related to recognition of tone of voice, facial expression, and body language don't work as expected in someone with autism. Now let's take a deeper look at this idea.

One brain, many specialized areas

At every given moment, our brain has a tremendous task: to keep us connected to the real world. This task includes processing sensory stimuli and deciding what information to discard and what information to pay attention to.

For example, to drive your car, your brain must keep an eye on the road, on the traffic signs, and on any other cars and obstacles.

Imagine you are on the road and the driver in front of you suddenly slams on the brakes. Maybe you were distracted, but once you see those braking lights turned on, what happens? Immediately your heart races, you begin to breathe faster, and your hands become cold and sweaty. But thanks to this sudden burst of energy, you can react in time, slow down your car and avoid hitting the other driver.

It all happened in an instant, but it required the processing of a tremendous amount of information. It was a simple action, slowing down your car, but it depended on a detailed coordination between your whole brain.

Let's take a closer look at this process. Once we are finished you'll have learned something fundamental about autism. Prepared?

Communication — the basis of mental processing

When the red lights of the front car lit up your brain had a chat with itself, asking questions and responding to each one of them. To simplify things, let us imagine that all the areas of your brain are video conferencing with one another:

Area dedicated to visual perception: "The red lights have lit up. What does that mean?"

Area responsible for comparing what is happening in the real world with our previous memories: "The front car will deaccelerate, if we continue at this speed we'll hit it".

Decision-Making Area: "What should we do? "

Area responsible for comparing what is happening in the real world with our previous memories: "We need to change direction or slow down. "

Decision-Making Area: "Which is the best option? "

Area responsible for comparing what is happening in the world real with our previous memories: "At this speed changing direction is more dangerous, we can lose control of the car. We are better off braking. "

Decision-Making Area: "How do we brake? "

Area responsible for comparing what's going on in the real world with our previous memories: " You have to press the center pedal with your right foot as hard as you can."

Decision-Making Area: "Roger that, I'm sending all this information to the conscious mind for prompt execution."

Now, from your point of view, what happened while you were driving your car?

You noticed the lights went on and, moments later, the idea of moving your right foot to the center pedal came into your conscious awareness. You just had to authorize that reaction.

But, take a closer look at the dialogue. We can imagine this same dialogue happening in a driving class.

The student is seating at the wheel for the first time. Although he is going very slowly, everything seems to grab his attention. While he is going at 20 mph the car in front of him brakes suddenly. "What now?" he asks his instructor. "Now you brake! Press the center pedal, fast!" the instructor replies.

Weeks later, he has his driver's license and is driving his own car. He no longer requires an instructor next to him, telling him what to do, but he still needs to process the information in a conscious way.

"Well, the car is slowing down, so I'd better slow down too," he thinks while pressing on the central pedal.

In these first few weeks after getting his license, he may need to focus so much on his driving to the point of being unable to hold a conversation with the other passengers in his car. But over time he will become more experienced.

A few months later and his brain is used to driving. He knows how to deal with entirely new situations. For example, he may have never dealt with an animal crossing the street. But when that happens he doesn't have to give it much thought. Immediately, a desire to brake arises in his conscious mind. This desire is so intense, so consuming, that he can't help but to brake as fast as he can.

But remember that first dialogue he had with his instructor? It's still present. It simply became automatic, unconscious.

Congratulations.

Now you have learned something fundamental about the autistic brain. What?

Well, you were not born with *any* area of your brain responsible for driving a car, were you? You had to learn to do it. At first, the process was exhausting. The first time you took the driver's seat everything was new.

You *depended* on your dialogue with your instructor. He told you what to do, how to do it, and when to do it.

"Now you need to shift gears. Press the left pedal with your left foot. While it is still down, move the shift lever back and to the left."

But, how would you feel if, instead of leading you step-by-step, the driving instructor simply said: "Let's go home"?

You would say, "But I never drove before. I do not even know how to start the car. **I need detailed instructions.**"

When we have to perform a task, and we have no area of our brain prepared from birth to perform this task, we need detailed instructions.

Do you remind the green-haired people with the syndrome we made up earlier? People with walks' syndrome had green hair, 4 toes on their right foot and were excellent drivers *from birth*.

These people are born with brains with several areas dedicated to driving. Scientists cannot understand why, but patients with Walks' syndrome have an area entirely dedicated to steering. Another area is prepared from birth to processing information regarding the use of the pedals, including the clutch. In addition, there are 2 areas dedicated to the use of the shift lever. It looks like magic, but when you put a person with Walks' syndrome in a car he looks like a fish inside water. He is at home. His hands and feet travel to all the right places. It's a fascinating thing to see. It seems like he's done this all his life.

Now imagine that someone with Walks' syndrome is trying to teach someone else to drive. How would their dialogue be? Let's see.

Person with Walks' syndrome: "Okay, now please, let's start the car and drive around the neighborhood."

Common person: "But how do I start the car?"

Person with Walks' syndrome: "What do you mean? You just turn the car on and that's it. "

And so, we came to the end of the illustration, for now. Maybe you haven't realized it yet, but you've learned more about autism than most people will learn in their lifetime. Let's look at the fundamental truths about autism that we have uncovered so far.

The autistic brain doesn't have the neurological connections related to empathy, interpretation of nonverbal language and socialization fully developed. For him, this is like driving a car for the first time. The difference is that this "car" has thousands of buttons and levers!

By comparison, those without autism know how to drive this car from birth.

Someone without autism is often called a neurotypical, that is, someone whose brain has a typical, or common, neurological configuration. A neurotypical has no idea of how this happens, but his "hands and feet," that is, his words, facial expressions, and body language simply "travel" to all the right places. He can make friends and understand people because his brain is able to process all the required information unconsciously, from birth.

Well, how can you help the autistic improve his social skills? Note the following dialog showing us how *not to* do this.

Neurotypical person: "Okay, now please try to make some friends at school."

Autistic person: "But, how do I make friends?"

Neurotypical person: "What do you mean? You just meet the people and befriend them."

Can you understand the frustration each of them must be feeling after this dialog?

The neurotypical person doesn't understand why such a straightforward task could be so difficult to execute. After all, it's so basic: "You get there, say hello to people and everything flows naturally."

In fact, even if the neurotypical person tried to, he'd have a hard time explaining everything, step by step. Why? Because social interaction comes naturally for him. His brain, through dozens of dedicated areas, can do countless processes at the unconscious level.

How can the neurotypical look at what his unconscious is doing and discern how to teach it step-by-step to someone who does not have those same areas? This is like asking an Englishman to teach his language to a Portuguese person. Where to start? Unless the Englishman is an English teacher this will be a very difficult task. For him, speaking English simply comes naturally.

On the other hand, for the autistic, the situation is no less frustrating. Depending on his degree of autism, the concept of making friends can be as complex as driving a state-of-the-art commercial airliner. When the autistic gets close to someone else it feels like they are entering the cockpit of the Boeing A320.

He keeps trying to remember what to do: "Okay, first I say, 'Hi, how are you?' then I wait for the answer and I say... I say what? "

The problem is even greater than that because, even if he memorizes everything he has to say, the truth is that social interactions are too unpredictable.

The person with autism says "Hi, how are you?" but his facial expression and tone of voice is somewhat off. It's like if he was in the cockpit of an airplane, holding the correct lever but pushing it too hard. Any good pilot would immediately realize he is a newbie. Likewise, the other children realize that something is not quite right in with the "Hi, how are you?"

How to help someone with autism?

We return to the example of the driving school. The instructor doesn't immediately teach you everything he knows about driving a car. Rather, he teaches you just the basics. You learn you can't let your car hit the other cars. You learn which foot corresponds to what pedal and some other simple rules. But it's only when you're on the road that you have a real sense of how everything works.

There you learn that when a car is blocking the road it may be necessary to violate the traffic code to some extent. For example, you may need to break the rule of never stepping on a continuous white line to avoid an obstacle.

These situations give the instructor an opportunity to teach you real-world applications of the driving code. A high number of these unique situations will provide you with a deeper learning experience.

Soon you will become able to understand what to do in an entirely new situation.

This is true **whenever you must perform a task for which you have no specialized area in your brain.**

We were not born with a brain set up to drive cars, change a burnt light bulb, or able to lay bricks and build walls.

In each of these cases, we need to be taught, step by step. This teaching must be very specific, simple and easy to understand. Then we try to do it by ourselves, and only then do we have a real sense of what is involved in the task. The more times we do it, the greater the number of different situations that. As we learn to deal with each of these new situations we increase our expertise in the task.

For example, if you have laid bricks for 30 years and have participated in the construction of all kinds of walls under all kinds of adverse conditions, you are well prepared to deal with any new situations that arise in your work. You are an expert.

In the beginning, this task required constant conscious effort: "Which brick should I grab first? How much mortar should I use? Where do I lay this brick? How hard should I press this new brick against the others?"

But 30 years later all this dialogue happens automatically in your mind. You don't even realize its there. If the wall starts bending to one side, you automatically know what to do. Even when an entirely new challenge arises, and you need to stop to think about how you will solve it, most processing takes place in the unconscious part of your mind.

It's true that you were *not born* with a brain area specialized in building walls, but over time, and with lots of hands-on experience you have developed a "pseudo-area". In what way? It turns out that the other areas with which you were born — such as motor coordination, abstract thinking, mathematical calculation, color and distance perception, among many others — have learned to work together to allow you to lay bricks like nobody else does.

That's exactly what happens in autism.

Whenever the autistic brain must perform a task for which he doesn't have a specialized area in his brain he needs to be taught step by step. These steps must be specific and simple, such as those found in an instruction manual for operating a washing machine. After all, this manual was written to help someone who has never used such a machine in their lives.

How do you teach anything to an autistic brain?

The more complex the task, the greater the need for simple, direct instructions.

Afterward, the autistic person needs a lot of opportunities to learn by trial and error, receiving feedback on how he can improve faster from his errors.

He needs someone skilled in the task helping him to understand that "the brick is not well laid." But that, by itself, is not enough. He also needs this specialist to tell him what he should have done to lay the brick correctly. This guidance must be given in simple and direct language.

It's true that there are many areas in the autistic brain that don't work well, but there are other areas working properly. In fact, some of them can even work *very* well. This means the instructions must be given in a way these areas understand.

For example, areas related to abstract thinking don't work well. Therefore, you need to talk in a concrete way. This is *vital*. It's the first step.

What is the difference between abstract and concrete language? How can you make sure you are talking with an autistic brain in a way he understands? The next chapter will explain this to us.

Chapter 3

The Difference Between Concrete and Abstract Thinking — The Secret to Communicating with Someone with Autism

An autistic person has many difficulties in processing abstract language. On the other hand, processing concrete language is actually very easy. So, if you want to talk to someone with moderate autism, such as Asperger's syndrome, you will be much more successful if you use concrete language.

If your goal is to communicate with someone with a deeper form of autism, bear in mind his or her communication centers may be almost completely inoperative. Even so, concrete language remains your best option.

What is *concrete* language?

Something concrete is something that you can point to. These are things that involve the senses. They can be seen, smelled, touched, heard or even, in some cases, savored.

And what about abstract language?

Note a few examples of abstract thinking:

- "Dogs are mammals."
- "We have to love one another."
- "It's good to be alive."

"Dogs are mammals."

A neurotypical person reads these sentences and immediately understands what they mean.

Someone with autism needs to convert these abstract ideas to something concrete and *only then* can he understand. This process is virtually automatic, but the point is that **this process of converting from concrete to abstract is present in those who have autism.**

"Dogs" and "mammals" are categories, not concrete things we can point to like bread, water, sun and so on.

Note this comment from someone with autism:

« In my case, to understand the abstract concept of "dogs", my brain immediately gives me images of various types of dogs. This is so instantaneous and fast that I need to be watchful to see it happening. The same is true for the word "mammals". As soon as I hear it, I immediately think about a very concrete image of a whale jumping and leaving behind a trail

> of splashing water, followed by an image containing many different animals from the mammal category, like seals, dolphins, bears, leopards and so forth. If I ask myself "what is a mammal?" My brain responds, "they are animals that drink milk when they are born." »

Did you notice the pattern? To understand the abstract concept of "mammal" this man with Asperger's syndrome required a tangible thing, such as an **image**, or **a definition of the word that used concrete ideas,** like drinking milk.

If this conversion fails to take place, the word "mammal" will have no meaning for the person with autism.

The more examples of members of a category — be it mammals, clothing, a subcategory like dogs, or any other category — the greater his understanding of the boundaries of that category.

Abstract thinking is an ability that develops from a very young age. When you hear the word "mammal" you immediately know what it is, without the need to access concrete things like "pictures" or "definitions with concrete explanations."

Upon learning about the difference between abstract and concrete thinking a young man with Asperger's said:

> « I had no idea that this [abstract thinking] existed. And frankly, I cannot quite understand how it's possible to understand something without resorting to concrete examples. »

For example, to understand the word "possible", notice how this same man described his mental processes:

> « Upon concentrating on the meaning of the word "possible" I see the image of someone throwing his hand. He is trying to catch something. If I want to understand what the word means more deeply, I get the image of someone jumping from the edge of a cliff, trying to get to the other side and actually being successful. Basically, my brain gives me several concrete images and videos to give me an idea of what the abstract concept represented by the word "possible" means. »

Not all the images that pop up in the autistic mind make sense to other people. Some are images mixed with feelings and they all come very quickly. But the point is that **their brain always needs to resort to something palpable that it already knows well** to understand abstract language.

It's as if the abstract concept were the roof and the concrete concepts were the walls, the pillars and all the remaining foundation that supports the roof.

"We have to love one another."

The same goes for the phrase "We have to love one another."

Again, we turn to someone with Asperger, who chose to remain anonymous, and asked him to describe the process for us:

> « For me, the expression "loving one another" means nothing. If you tell me "you have to love me" I don't know what you mean. Then, the image of one person embracing another, of one person offering something to another, along with a feeling in my body, automatically appears in my mind. »

What is "love"? It is only after combining all these concrete images that the autistic brain can come to a conclusion.

However, this conclusion happens only within the sphere of concrete examples that the autistic person knows.

The more concrete examples he has, the greater his understanding of the concept and the greater his ability to perceive whether an entirely new action falls within the category of "loving others."

For example, we ask this person: "Is shaking hands part of 'loving others?'" Note the fascinating explanation:

> « When I think of shaking hands and in love, the image of two people appears in my mind. They are wearing a suit and a combining tie, they are shaking hands and smiling. One puts his hand on the other's shoulder. You can see they are good friends. So, yes, shaking hands can be a part of loving others. »

The neurotypical person doesn't need this intermediate step because his brain can understand what "loving one another" means.

"It's good to be alive."

« Likewise, the expression "It's good to be alive." brings up in my mind the image of someone sitting, smiling. Then, the camera focuses on his breathing. The person is smiling, with his eyes closed, while taking a deep breath. If I want to understand the meaning of the individual words used in the phrase, "good" makes me think of the image of someone smiling. "Alive" makes a little movie of someone breathing appear. If I think more about the meaning of "alive" the image of someone in a coffin appears along with a commentary saying: "It's the opposite of this". »

These concrete examples are variable. It doesn't mean that these specific images and videos will always appear, but *something* concrete will take place in the autistic brain.

The point is always the same: the autistic brain only understands abstract concepts if it has *sufficient* concrete examples illustrating the concept. The more concrete examples the autistic person has, the greater his understanding of the meaning of the abstract concept communicated to him.

This means that the best way to teach someone with autism is to present an image or story and say, "this is an example of "x".

At the end of many examples of "x", the autistic will understand the meaning of "x". How the person will know that the autistic really understands the meaning of "x"? When he is able to formulate his own entirely new examples of "x".

Let's look at a concrete example of this abstract explanation.

What is an abstract concept?

All abstract concepts have a list of rules of what belongs to this concept and what doesn't.

These rules are written in a concrete way. Or, when they are not, they are written in an abstract language that is closer to the concrete. It's like an onion. You have several layers of abstraction.

For example, note the word "mammals." Some rules are:

- They are vertebrates.
- They have mammary glands that, in females, produce milk for feeding their babies.
- They have fur, except dolphins and some whales, which only have embryonic hair.
- Their heart has four chambers.

Looking at the last feature, "Their heart has four chambers", this expression is far less abstract than "mammals."

Again, we turn to someone with autism to tell us how the autistic brain works:

> « I can easily imagine a heart with four divisions. Although the word "chambers" is abstract. To understand it I imagine the pyramids with their many chambers or divisions, and then the concept is clear: a heart with four little rooms. »

On the other hand, "mammary glands" is much more concrete.

> « I think of a cow, with her mammary glands. It's the first image that pops up in my mind. »

What's the lesson for us?

To communicate with someone with autism, give him as many examples as you can. Use concrete language in these examples. Then ask him to create his own examples. If he cannot create entirely new examples it's because he hasn't yet fully understood the abstract concept you are trying to convey to him.

However, when he understands, you will be amazed at the mental fluidity with which he can connect this new understanding with everything else he already knows and with how he becomes capable of creating new ideas.

How can you train yourself to explain something abstract in a concrete way?

Imagine you were forbidden to speak or write. How would you explain an abstract idea?

Imagine explaining the meaning of the word "mammal" without being able to speak or write. How would you do it?

Maybe mimicking. In that case, what gestures would you use? To where would you point? What would you draw on a piece of paper?

Surely you would draw animals. But if you just drew 3 or 4 animals, would that be sufficient for the person to understand you were referring to "mammals" and not, for example, to the abstract concept of "animals"?

Maybe you would end up drawing other animals that are not mammals like birds or fish and put an "X" on them to show that they are out.

In fact, you'd be like saying:

"Look, these are the limits of the abstract concept I want to teach you. "Whale, dog, and cat are within limits. This sardine, this eagle and this toad are outside the boundaries."

But even then, that would not be enough to clearly define the boundaries of the concept of a "mammal." You would need more animals, many more. Tens or hundreds of sketches on a sheet of paper of many different types of animals. The more examples of animals you gave, the greater the understanding of what you were trying to describe.

It would come to a point when the other person would be able to see which animals are in the category and which animals are not, even if you hadn't literally told them you were talking about "mammals."

Now try to do the same with even more abstract ideas such as explaining the concept of "category" or explaining the meaning of "abstract" or even explaining the concept of "example" and the very word "concept"! It becomes increasingly complicated to do so without being able to speak or write, don't you agree?

On the other hand, if you lower the level of abstraction and try to explain simpler abstract words like "clothing," "food," "dogs," or "books," your task becomes easier.

So, start with the concrete and slowly, use the concrete words the autistic person already knows to teach him slightly more abstract things.

Use pictures from the Internet or magazines, draw pictures or show him objects to teach him any concrete concepts. Then, use these same concrete examples as stepping stones for teaching him increasingly abstract concepts. Bit by bit, these examples will allow his own brain to understand spoken and written language better.

This means you'll be teaching "cat" by point to images of cats and repeating "cat" aloud every time. When your child can point to entirely new images of cats and systematically identify them, you'll know he understands. Then you can teach him a new concept.

The deeper the level of autism, the greater your challenge. Some autistics may even take a long time to learn some basic words. But do not give up! Your effort will be rewarded.

Alternatively, if you are dealing with someone with a more moderate form of autism and who already has a good mastery of spoken language, as someone with Asperger's syndrome, what things should you teach?

You should focus your efforts on helping him to assimilate more complex abstract concepts related to the areas in which he has the most difficulty.

In the next chapter, we will analyze one of the areas in which the Autistic child needs the most help: the development of Emotional Intelligence.

We will look at each of the fundamental human emotions and try to understand how to apply what we have just learned about concrete thinking and abstract thinking, to help the autistic person to deepen their ability to deal with emotions.

Although the following instructions are especially useful for those who can communicate, the basic principles will apply to any type of autism.

Chapter 4

Emotional Intelligence for the Autistic — yes, it's possible for someone with autism to understand emotions

This chapter was prepared to teach something very abstract, emotional intelligence, in a concrete way. This means that to educate someone with autism, you can adapt the chapter itself. Adapt the examples to the age and level of understanding of the person you are teaching.

At the same time, if you have autism, this chapter will help you to significantly increase your own emotional intelligence.

In fact, even someone *without autism* will benefit from the information contained here because it's universal.

Where to start?

We start with the brain. In our brain, we have specific areas evaluating the state of our *resources* and our *needs.*

When there is a change in either of these, our body *warns us* and *modifies itself* to help us deal with this change.

Confused by these two phrases? Don't worry. The following examples will make the point clear. Then we'll talk about how it all relates to autism.

Needs

We all have the same human needs. These needs include:

- **Eating**

- **Drinking water**

- **Sleeping**

- **Resting** (like when we sit down for a while to recover our energy)

- **Breathing**

- **Having our bodies at the right temperature**

- **Being away from things that cause us pain**

- **Excretion**

And to meet these needs we use *resources.*

Resources

A resource is everything that makes it possible to satisfy a need. For example, to satisfy the need to **eat** we can use various resources such as bread, meat, rice, fruit, vegetables and so on.

To satisfy the need to **drink water** we need a very specific and irreplaceable resource: water.

As for the need to **sleep**, we just need to have access to a place that is comfortable enough to allow our body to shut down and sleep peacefully. To **rest,** we require a place where we can sit for a while.

When it comes to **breathing** we need another resource that can't be replaced: air with the correct concentration of gases.

To keep our body at the **correct temperature** we have a variety of resources at our disposal, such as a house, clothes, air conditioning, fans, heaters and many other means of modifying our temperature.

Being **away from pain** requires access to more specific resources such as a doctor, medication, or specific information on how to act to relieve any pain that we are feeling. But in its most basic form, we just need to have enough space to move away from anything that can cause us suffering.

The need for **excretion** involves resources such as adequate sanitation facilities, or at the very least: an open field.

These are some of the basic *needs* we all have. And we use *resources* to satisfy them. Beyond these, there are other, more abstract needs that we will discuss shortly.

Emotions

What happens when our needs are not being met? At least two things will take place:

1. Our body will warn us through sensations.

2. Our brain will fill our conscious mind with suggestions about what to do next.

1. Our body warns us through sensations

There are areas of our brain responsible for checking how our needs are. The way they do this is very complex and involves hormones, electrical signals and the interaction between the brain and our various organs.

For example, for a sensation such as hunger to arise, the following occurs:

1. Our brain is always communicating with the stomach and the other organs. Eventually, the brain will receive the following message: "We need more food." All this communication happens without our knowledge. It's an unconscious process.

2. When the unconscious part of the brain sends a message to the conscious part, the person, who was minding his own business, feels hungry. His mind was full of thoughts about the work he was doing, but now he is thinking more and more about food.

   The more our body believes we need to eat, the greater the hunger it makes us feel, and the greater the number of thoughts about food crossing our mind.

The same goes for the other needs:

- **Food** ⇒ We feel hungry.

- **Water intake** ⇒ We feel thirsty.

- **Sleeping** ⇒ We feel sleepy.

- **Rest** ⇒ We feel tired.

- **Breathing** ⇒ If we are unable to breathe, like when we are underwater, we feel an increasing distress to inspire.

- **Have our body at the right temperature** ⇒ We feel discomfort.

- **Being away from things that cause us pain** ⇒ We will feel pain if we ignore the requirements of this need.

- **Excretion** ⇒ A desire to urinate or defecate.

2. Our brain will fill our conscious mind with suggestions about what to do next.

When we were babies, our brain learned what resources can be used to meet our needs. So, when we are thirsty we think of water, not food.

- **Food** ⇒ We think more and more about food.

- **Water intake** ⇒ We think about drinking water.

- **Sleeping** ⇒ We keep thinking about how good it would be to lay down on our bed.

- **Resting** ⇒ Thoughts about how good sitting down would feel keeping popping up in our mind.

- **Breathing** ⇒ When this need needs to be met we can't think of anything else. Our whole focus is on finding a way to breathe.

- **Having our body at the right temperature** ⇒ If we are cold, ideas about how to warm us come up in our head. If it's too hot, we can only think about taking off our clothes or in a cold shower.

- **Being away from things that cause us pain** ⇒ When we touch something that causes us pain, our immediate reaction is to back off. Our mind becomes filled with ideas on how to escape. If we believe something can harm us, we can only think about getting away from it.

- **Excretion** ⇒ We only think about the toilet. If the need is too great, bolder ideas appear in our mind, like urinating behind a bush.

Now let's get into the abstract part. Prepared?

- Depending on what we **believe** about the *availability of the resources* we use to meet our needs, we will feel an **emotion**.

In a moment we analyze in depth the meaning of this phrase. First, however, it's necessary to talk about these emotions our body makes us feel.

There are many different words to describe emotions. Despite this, experts such as Paul Ekman agree that there are only a small number of basic emotions. These emotions can blend with each other and with sensations to form more complex emotions.

What are our basic, or primary, emotions?

1. Happiness

2. Fear

3. Anger

4. Disgust

5. Surprise

6. Sadness

Let us now analyze each one of them. Don't despair. In a few minutes, everything will make perfect sense. Before you know it, you will be in possession of the kind of concrete information that changes lives. This will allow you to understand and explain, in a simple way, all this abstract world of needs, resources, and emotions.

See if you can you spot the pattern.

Understanding the Emotions: Happiness

We feel happy when we **believe** we have access to a resource that can meet a need and afterward when we actually use it to satisfy our need.

Examples:

- I'm hungry. Then I remember the mouthwatering dish my wife has prepared for me. I feel **happy**. I get home, I smell the food. My expectation that my need will soon be met increases. My **happiness** is higher. I sit down at the table and begin to eat. I finish the meal and feel satisfied. This kind of *satisfaction* is the **happiness** we are talking about. It's more than a simple moment of joy or laughter. More examples follow.

- I'm sleepy. I start thinking that at the end of the day I will have a very comfortable bed where I will be able to lie down: I feel **happy**. When it's time to go to sleep, I lie down. When I wake up I feel **happy**, because I satisfied my need to sleep.

- The same happens when we breathe deeply or when we finally stop feeling some pain we had.

- When we get cold and wrap ourselves in a cozy blanket or when it's hot and we enter a room with air conditioning.

- When we are tired and finally sit down.

- When we are in real need of going to the bathroom, but it's occupied. Suddenly the door opens, and we can get inside. We feel happy.

Happiness exists in degrees. **The greater my certainty that my need will really be satisfied, the greater my degree of happiness.** After considering the remaining emotions, we will talk more about degrees.

What is the purpose of happiness?

happiness is a motivating force. It makes us **want to use** the resources that fulfill our needs and it's a **reward** that our body gives us when we meet our needs. Next time we'll want to use that resource to meet our needs even more.

Understanding Emotions: Fear

We experience fear when we **believe that something bad will happen to a resource** that meets a need. This expectation that something bad will happen causes many changes in our body.

These changes cause sensations. We call this set of changes and sensations "fear."

For example, imagine that my boss calls me, asking me to meet him in his office. His voice is tense and irritated. I begin to think about the mistakes I made last week. Am I going to be lectured? Will I get fired?

The **more I believe** in these outcomes, the **greater my fear.**

But why am I afraid? Because I believe I need my job to have access to the resources that satisfy my needs. I believe that my job gives me money, which in turn gives me access to food and other important things.

This job also increases the value I think I have. Losing my job means losing that value. Why is value so important? It's interesting that in ancient Greek, the word "value" was linked with the concept of "weight." The less "value" I have in front of other people's the lesser the "weight" my needs will have for them. When they make decisions, I will have less power to influence these decisions and to deal with them.

Then, faced with the possibility of losing my job, my brain keeps thinking over all these possibilities. The feelings and sensations we call "fear" are the result of this thinking process.

Another example involves health. If I start having chest pains I may end up going to google to search for "heart attack symptoms." Then, I begin to read about the symptoms of an imminent heart attack, "chest pain, fatigue, difficulty breathing." The result? The more I believe that I am having a heart attack, the greater my fear.

In these examples, it seems fear isn't useful. After all, how does fear protect me from being fired? How does fear protect me from having a heart attack?

The truth, however, is that fear is quite helpful. Fear is for protection. When we are afraid we are alert, we are careful, and we are much more motivated to make decisions that protect us.

For example, if I feel confident, I will speak to my boss in a completely different way than if I am feeling scared. Fear will help me to be careful, to acknowledge that I have made a mistake and to apologize.

The same happens with the symptoms of a heart attack. Fear will cause me to do something about it. Whether it's calling 911 or driving to the hospital.

As the last example, imagine that you are walking down the street and a dog appears. This dog is big, and it's barking at you. He begins to move toward you while growling. You don't know how to react, so your brain makes some swift calculations: "This dog is dangerous, if it attacks me I'll end up badly hurt." The more you believe that (1) you can be attacked and that (2) this attack will harm you, the greater your fear. The greater your fear the higher your focus in doing the best you can to protect yourself.

Now, depending on what you believe to be the right thing to do, fear may motivate you to stand still, paralyzed without moving, to flee into some yard or even to attack the dog!

What is the purpose of fear?

Fear is the name given to the sensations we feel in our body when our brain detects a threat. Fear guarantees that we won't ignore this threat and that we will do everything we can to survive it. The action we will end up taking depends on our beliefs about the situation.

Understanding Emotions: Anger

For me, anger is one of the most fascinating emotions. It arises when we **believe that an injustice has occurred.** The need for justice is so important to us that we have a whole emotion designed to deal with any attack on what we believe to be fair.

Anger is a very powerful emotion. When our brain detects an injustice, it sends out several hormones, or messengers, that modify us completely. In what way?

Our conscious mind is filled with thoughts about how the injustice could be corrected. We feel our hearts beating hard, our breathing increases, and our muscles tense up. Why is this happening? Because our brain is turning our whole body into a war machine.

Anger, when left uncontrolled is a devastating emotion. It can lead us to do things we end up regretting a lot, once anger decreases.

However, in itself, anger isn't evil.

Like fear, anger is an emotion that **drives us to action.** Unfortunately, the degree of anger can be so great that it becomes difficult to control. Think of anger like a fast car. The higher your speed the longer it takes to brake and change direction. Similarly, when we are very angry it's difficult to steer away from violent thoughts. All because our brain detected an injustice.

What is an injustice?

"Injustice" is an abstract word. How can we transform it into something more concrete? Imagine a judge. The judge's work is closely linked to justice.

When a case is brought to court the judge makes a **comparison**. The judge compares what **should have happened** to what **actually happened**. Then, the judge decides *what must be done* to correct things. To make that decision the judge considers the *intent* of the person who has done the wrong action.

For example, if an elderly lady is walking down the street and drops her wallet without noticing, how should other people react? The right thing to do is to pick up the, call the lady and give her back the wallet. This means that if a man picks up the wallet and hides it in his pocket, he is doing something wrong.

When faced with this situation the judge compares what *was done* — stealing the wallet — with what *should* have been done: returning the wallet.

If the wallet had been returned, the judge would have decided that the action had been fair. The judge would feel happy, he would praise the man for his integrity. But the wallet was stolen. This is an injustice. It shouldn't have happened. The judge feels angry and with the need to reestablish justice.

Then, this judge will deliberate on an appropriate course of action. He may decide the lady has the right to be compensated for the loss of money and all the anxiety she went through. He may also decide to punish the thief for his wrongdoing.

However, before coming up with his final decision, the judge will also consider the *intention* of the man. This can change everything.

For example, suppose several eyewitnesses testify to the fact that the man was about to return the wallet, but didn't do so due to circumstances beyond his control. In this case, even though what was done remains the same, the judge's opinion changes. Once the judge realizes the man's intentions weren't bad, he stops feeling angry. Perhaps he is now sad, as he considers all the unnecessary emotional turmoil this whole situation has caused both to the man and to the old lady.

In the same way, our brain has a long list of rules detailing what we believe to be right and wrong.

We may not think about it much, but the human being has a strong need for justice. This is observed early in children. For example, they find it unfair if their schoolmate gets a bigger slice of cake than they did.

It's also interesting to consider how even a thief has a sense of justice. The thief *doesn't like* to be robbed. He gets angry. His brain keeps telling him, "It's not fair!" And he gets angry at the person who stole something from him.

Anger drives action. In the case of the child, he may cry or demand an explanation, "Why is his slice bigger than mine?" In the case of the thief, he may orchestrate a plan to get his revenge.

Anger is this inner force that leads us to do something to correct what we believe was unfair. This force comes about whenever our brain, like a judge, compares what happened to what our internal rules say should have happened. If a difference is detected between these two things, and if we believe that the other person acted with a bad intention, we create an image of an enemy in our mind. We get angry.

Sometimes we can even get angry at ourselves. This happens when we realize that we have done something we shouldn't have done. Although, in these cases, we don't normally use a word as strong as "anger." We use other expressions such as "I am annoyed with myself" or "I'm so frustrated with me." However, all these expressions refer to the same emotion, in greater or lesser degree, anger.

What is the purpose of anger?

Anger causes us to become impatient. We want to *act now* and make things right again. Unfortunately, anger is blind. It moves us to act, but it doesn't tell us how to act. Someone with bad principles or with little self-control can end up harming someone else. But when used properly, anger can motivate us to act in a constructive way.

For example, if I watch a lady being robbed, anger will make me want to do something about it to help the lady. For example, I may call the police and wait near the lady, trying to calm her down, until the police officers arrive. I felt outraged, or angry, and this strong emotion kept me from being indifferent and doing nothing.

Understanding Emotions: Disgust

One of the most important resources we have is our physical and mental energy. That is why our brain is designed to make us **want to move away from anything that might wear us out physically or mentally.**

For example, what if I ask you to make some calculations?

Take the test:

- $1 + 1 = ?$

- $3 + 5 = ?$

- $24 + 65 = ?$

- $55 + 15 = ?$

- $9 \times 78 = ?$

- $1849 \times 4 = ?$

- $354651 - 456651 = ?$

- $2375 / 51 = ?$

Did you notice it? As the problems became increasingly complex, your brain began to reject solving them. It made you feel *disgusted.* Unless, of course, you have a lot of mental energy available. If so, continue to solve complex problems. Soon, your body will warn you about the loss of mental energy. In what way?

Unless you love arithmetic, your stomach will tighten a little, your muscles will tense up, and, if you hate math, you may even feel a certain level of nausea, This is the feeling of disgust and is one of our primary emotions.

We are used to associating disgust with the smell of rotten food or with the sight of a disturbing image. However, disgust is a much more general protection mechanism.

All the time, our unconscious mind must decide whether a stimulus is too much for us or not, and if it is, **our body is modified to make it easier to reject that same stimulus**. How can we exemplify this?

Again, spoiled food provides us with a familiar example. As soon as you smell the rotten odor you can easily feel your body constrict and your digestive system changing to promote *expulsion* of food, rather than preparing you to digest it.

What we often don't realize is that other people, or even things, can provoke that same emotion in us. What happens is that, just as our body has difficulty digesting spoiled food, our minds also have difficulty processing an interaction with a difficult person.

Complicated people are exhausting to our psyche. No wonder then, that the mere thought of spending an afternoon with one of these people can contract our whole body. It is as if our mind was telling us that it refuses to deal with that person with the same intensity that our digestive system refuses to digest spoiled food

Sometimes being tired is all that is needed. When we are tired, even the thought of solving 41 + 27 can be enough to cause our stomach to contract in disgust.

Can you remember a time when you didn't feel like seeing anyone? Maybe you were sleepy or maybe you just felt tired after a hard day of work. At times like these, even the idea of dealing with a loved one can cause a certain level of disgust.

At those times, it's like as if our brain kept telling us, "I refuse to process more information! I want to rest! "

The more we believe that something will wear us down, the greater the disgust we'll feel.

What is the purpose of disgust?

Disgust gives us the strength to reject things that wear us down or harm us. It's just a protection mechanism. It motivates us to move away from those types of stimuli.

Understanding Emotions: Surprise

Our brain is very fast. All the time it processes a vast amount of information. However, our brain is not infinitely fast.

Imagine you are about to open the door and enter your home after a day of work. In these final moments, when you are unlocking the door, your brain is working hard to assist you. In your mind, details about what you need to do next pop up. You imagine yourself stepping inside, turning on the lights, placing your keys and coat in the right place, and walking to the bathroom to wash your hands and refresh your face.

That way, when you finish rolling the key and unlocking the door, all these actions will flow smoothly, almost automatically. You don't need to waste mental energy. Home is your mental refuge, your source of relaxation. But...

Imagine that when you turn on the light you are faced with a complete mess. Everything is turned upside down. The drawers are open. The furniture is all over the place. Clothes and papers are scattered across the floor. What do you think? How do you feel?

For a few moments, you stand still. Processing all that you have just observed.

The situation you came across is **so different from what you expected** that your brain **can't process everything in real time.** It takes a few seconds. You're feeling *surprised.*

Surprise is an emotion that occurs when what happens is very different from what we had anticipated. At that time, our brain and body are modified to facilitate the processing of that new and unexpected situation.

Note a few examples:

- Your cell phone rings while you are absorbed in a task and for a moment you become paralyzed, changing the "disk" in your brain.

- You cross the road at the same time that you wonder what you'll do when you get to the store. Suddenly you hear the screeching sound of rubber fighting asphalt. Your body is paralyzed for a moment while your brain processes what is happening, "a car is coming our way, what do I need to do? Should I stand still? Do I run or jump? What's the best option?" And then you finally wake up and run to the other side of the road.

- You're talking to your wife and suddenly her face becomes pale. You stand there, paralyzed for a moment. "What happened?" you finally mumble, "Are you okay?"

- You are in a foreign country and suddenly, from the crowd, someone says your name.

All these examples highlight the key point: when our brain needs to process something unexpected, that it deems urgent, it puts all other mental processes on hold.

We may even say that, in a way, surprise is a "pre-emotion" because it occurs before other emotions. It is **the instant before our brain decides how it should react.**

But sometimes, this moment of surprise lasts more than a few seconds.

Back to our example, after staring at the mess in your house for a few moments, you finally finish processing that unexpected situation. "I've been robbed."

What will you feel next? It depends. If you believe the thieves may still be inside your home or if you think there's a strong likelihood of being robbed again, you will experience fear. Also anger, as you realize the tremendous injustice of the situation. You may even feel severe pain in your stomach as your mind realizes just how inconceivable this is. In this latter case, you'd be feeling a strong form of disgust.

"Call the police, check everything to see what was stolen, mourn all that was lots, deal with the fear of being robbed again" — all this is too much to process.

Under this trialing circumstances, some people may even end up literally vomiting from disgust.

What is the purpose of surprise?

Surprise modifies our body to **process information faster**. We stand still, our previous thoughts waiting in the background. Our body is on standby, ready to react to the situation as soon as the brain processes it just enough.

Meanwhile, the brain assesses how the new situation affects our resources and the needs they met, and then decides what the next most appropriate emotion is.

Understanding Emotions: Sadness

Sadness is intimately connected with **loss.** For example, people are a resource that meets our needs. Maybe this sentence sounds cold to you. If this is the case note the following: One of the most important needs that human beings have is to **contribute to the wellbeing of others.** Other people allow us to do this. In this way, they become a *resource* that allows us to satisfy our need to contribute to their well-being.

For example, let's talk about happiness again. Happiness is felt when we meet our needs. It's how our brain rewards us when we meet our own needs. Now the question is: What makes us happier, meeting *our own* needs or meeting the needs of *others?*

Imagine the following situations:

- I have a loaf of bread. In front of me is a hungry child. I can even see his ribs silhouette. Well, I may be hungry. Eating bread would satisfy my need and give me some measure of satisfaction. But how would I feel if I ate the bread while that hungry child stares at me? Would I be truly happy? On the other hand, if I gave the child all the bread, how would I feel? My degree of joy will be so high that I may end up with tears streaming down my face.

- Some videos recorded by security cameras in train stations show people who inadvertently, or for some other reason, fall into the train tracks. Often, how do other people react? They risk their lives by jumping to the line and helping the other person get out of there. How do they feel when they think about what they did? Happy, satisfied.

- A parent who loves their child volunteers to transplant an organ, such as a kidney or a portion of his liver.

The more we love our neighbor, the easier it becomes to put their needs ahead of our own. And when we do that we feel great satisfaction.

In this way, others become a resource to satisfy our needs.

Then, as you can imagine, when we lose this resource, this is very traumatic. When someone we love dies, we can no longer contribute to that person's well-being. In this way, our life loses a portion of its meaning. How big is that portion? It depends.

In the case of the loss of a close relative, such as a child, a parent, a beloved grandpa or spouse, the loss is overwhelming. It takes many years to recover completely. Sometimes, this recovery is never complete, because what has been lost is irreplaceable.

The same can happen when we lose a treasured pet or when we lose our health. These are very large losses, difficult to overcome.

Other losses are smaller. If I really like an object, maybe something that was offered to me by a friend or something that is very useful, how do I feel when I lose it? I'm sad, of course.

The same thing happens when we lose something abstract. Going back to the employment example. My job made me feel valued. Now that I've lost it, I start to believe that others will give me less value. My opinions and my needs will have less weight in their decisions. I feel afraid, but I also feel sadness. This sadness is linked to my perceived loss of something abstract: value.

Sadness is like this, a testimony of how important what we lost was for us.

It's difficult to deal with sadness. First, we need to give our brains time to process what happened and the changes that will take place in our lives now that we no longer have this lost resource. Then, we need to find other resources that will allow us to meet the needs that were being met by what was lost. This time to process things, and this pursuit of other resources that meet our needs, will mitigate the grief caused by the loss.

What is the purpose of sadness?

Sadness helps us deal with loss. Feelings of sadness make sure we **take the time needed to process** the meaning of our loss. It's as if our brain had to take a few days off from everything else to rearrange everything relating to what was lost. Sadness is a way for our brain to help us **recognize the importance of what was lost**. It prevents us from being indifferent.

In addition, sadness promotes reactions that motivate others to help us. The greater the sadness the greater the crying, the facial expressions expressing pain, and the changes in our tone of voice and body language. All this stimulates compassion in others along with a desire to help. It's as if, **by bringing about these changes in our behavior, our brain was recruiting other brains to help us process the loss**.

Just thinking about losing someone, or something, we love, is enough to make us feel sad. This moves us to **care and love even more and to further protect** this resource.

Just like any other emotion, sadness shouldn't be thought of as a bad thing. It's just the right reaction to deal with the loss of something, or someone, important.

How does someone with autism deal with emotions?

Summarizing, so far, we've learned that:

- **Happiness** is felt when we use a resource to fulfill a need. Whether it's our own need or someone else's need.

- **Fear** arises when our brain predicts that a resource that meets our needs is in danger of being damaged or lost.

- **Anger** is felt when our need for justice is disturbed.

- **Disgust** occurs when something, or someone, wear us down and drains our mental or physical energy.

- **Surprise** happens in response to an unexpected stimulus.

- **Sadness** results from losing a resource. It's a coping mechanism.

People with autism have processing difficulties in the areas of the brain responsible for emotional processing. This means they don't always realize what they are feeling, why they are feeling it and what they should do next.

How does this work in practice?

Note the difference in the following examples.

First, imagine that a young neurotypical child — that is, one who doesn't have autism — lost his favorite toy. What happens next?

1. His brain registers the loss.

2. His brain orders the modification of the organism to facilitate processing the loss: the young man feels these new sensations as sadness.

3. This sadness is accompanied by a strong desire to get up and look for his loved ones. His brain recognizes other people as a source of support. His brain also initiates the crying mechanism, because it knows this will signal his distress to the other brains and recruit their help.

4. At the same time, the young child feels fear. How will things change now that favorite toy is gone? This makes his stomach to contract and he becomes ever more distressed.

5. His brain creates in him the need to share these fears with his mother.

6. At the same time, the young man is feeling angry too. "How could I be so silly and lose my bear?" He says aloud. This allows his mother to understand what is going on in the boy's mind. With her wisdom and trough comforting words and gestures, she can help him cope with his loss.

Now, let's Imagine a young man with autism going through the same situation:

1. His brain registers the loss.

2. Communication between the areas processing the loss and the rest of the brain is incomplete.

3. The young man feels an upset stomach but fails to associate this disturbing sensation with neither sadness nor fear.

4. He may even recognize that he needs support, but his body feels disgusted at the thought of reaching out for help. This happens because social interaction tends to be exhausting to his psyche. This is especially true now that he is dealing with all these unpleasant sensations in his body.

5. He is now quiet, locked inside himself. He feels angry but doesn't quite understand why and is unable to verbalize the distressing images and thoughts crossing through his mind.

6. His mother notices this change in behavior and approaches him, trying to understand what's wrong. But the young man can't explain what's happening to him.

7. He tries to cry but may end up yelling or making other sounds, depending on the degree of his autism. After all,

several areas of his brain are failing to communicate properly with each other at this critical moment.

8. The distress he feels inside is so great that he becomes restless, rocking in his seat and fidgeting.

9. His mother tries to hug him to comfort him, but he rejects the hug. To his overwhelmed brain, any physical contact is seen as one more extra thing to process.

10. The mother steps back. Disheartened at the sight of her son humming and flapping his hands.

11. Sometime later, he slowly begins to calm down.

We will soon understand exactly what happened in steps 8, 9, and 10. However, everything we have learned so far, about how the autistic brain works and how it processes emotions, is enough for us to understand why this young man reacted so differently from the neurotypical boy.

As you can imagine, forcing the young autistic boy to explain what's wrong, can easily be met with impoliteness. Someone with no knowledge of autism might conclude, "This young man is rude and aggressive."

But an insightful understand person sees things more deeply, "Right now. this young man is dealing with strong feelings and distressing thoughts. These cause him many sensations his brain is unable to process at this time. I'll let him rest for now and I'll try to engage him at a later time."

From now on, you, the reader, belong to this elite of insightful people who can understand things more deeply. Use this knowledge to educate others.

Several emotions can occur together and in degrees

In addition to the struggle to understand what emotions are — since they are so abstract — and the trouble in realizing what one is feeling, someone with autism must deal with yet another obstacle. One extra difficulty of autism has to do with the *degree* of your emotional reactions.

For example, imagine that the whole family agreed to go visit a museum this weekend. Saturday morning, the child with Asperger is looking forward to the trip, just like the whole family. Then, due to an unforeseen issue, the family is unable to make the trip. Everyone is disappointed but the child with Asperger reacts as if it were the end of the world.

It looks like as if there was only "black" or "white" without shades of gray. Either everything is fine, or it's the end of the world. From zero to 10 it seems that the level of sadness, anger or fear is either at 0 or 10, without passing through any of the intermediate values.

Moreover, the person with autism has difficulty understanding what emotion he is feeling, except when it's already present at a very high degree.

This can be caused by problems related to the area responsible for detecting the contraction of the stomach, or by an inability to associate the contraction of the stomach with an external stimulus.

It's as if there's a plate of spoiled food in front of me and I'm feeling disgusted. However, my brain doesn't make the connection and I fail to link the disgust I'm feeling with the spoiled food. Because of this, I continue to eat the rotten food. Then, when I'm already nauseated, I realize everything, "It was the food!"

Why does this happen?

There are essentially two possible reasons: Either the responsible areas are not working well, or they are working properly but the "cables" linking them to the rest of the brain are improperly connected. Therefore, the message doesn't get through. The complete picture never reaches the conscious mind, until it's too late.

In the same way, a neurotypical person can do the opposite. After feeling fear, he can calm himself down. Conversely, an autistic person has a lot more difficulties doing this. As much as his conscious mind wishes to calm down, it seems that this command information is never sent to where it should.

It's common for someone with autism to have a harder time controlling his or her temperament. He seems to explode even when he didn't want to. This the so-called *meltdown* we'll cover later.

For now, however, our question is: How to apply this concrete understanding of what emotions are in a way that helps both the autistic person and their family? Let's see.

Practical emotional intelligence for the autistic

The concept of emotional intelligence is abstract. To make it more concrete we will divide it into 2 main concepts:

1. Being able to identify any emotions being felt and the situations triggering them. This involves identifying emotions by name and understanding the kind of situations that usually cause them.

   Example: Recognizing that suffering an injustice usually triggers anger, or that going through a loss leads to sadness.

2. Being able to modulate, or control, emotions; either in ourselves or in other people.

   Example: Being able to calm yourself down when you are scared or angry and being able to comfort someone who is sad.

Now, we'll be looking at how to apply what we have learned so far to each of these areas.

Identifying and dealing with Happiness

How can you identify happiness?

Happiness means more than laughing. It's characterized by a pleasant sensation in our body. When we are feeling this kind of enjoyable feeling we can ask ourselves:

- Did I meet my needs?

- Did I contribute to someone else's well-being?

- Has anything strengthened my self-esteem?

- Did I receive any compliment?

- Did I meet a basic need like sleeping, eating or resting?

- Do I believe something positive will happen soon? What?

How does happiness affect us?

Happiness creates in us a desire to share our ideas and experiences with others. We feel a natural curiosity and a willingness to explore the environment around us and interact with others — even if we have social difficulties or autism. A happy person with Asperger's will gladly speak at length with someone else about his favorite topic. Also, someone with a deeper kind of autism, when happy, will make attempts at interaction with the outside. For example, if hungry, the smell of a favorite food can produce a desire to interact with the outside world.

What can make someone happy?

We make ourselves happy whenever we, *willingly,* do something in favor of another person — for it satisfies our innate need to contribute to the wellbeing of others — or when we, or another person, fulfill any of our many needs.

We feel happy to the same degree that our needs are being met.

Moreover, the very expectation and belief that our needs will soon be met make us happy.

In this sense "happiness" is synonymous both with "satisfaction" and with "hope".

The "negative" emotions

In the following pages, we will analyze the so-called "negative" emotions. Not that they are bad in themselves, it's just that they are usually associated with sensations that we don't like to feel for a long time. These include a tight stomach, tingling sensations, muscle tension, and changes in heart rhythm and breathing rate.

Moreover, the fact that they have in *common* all these characteristics makes it difficult to identify them. How can we solve this problem? We need to look beyond sensations.

As such, we will focus on another aspect:

- The relationship between **each of these emotions** and (1) our **needs** and (2) the **resources** our brain believes it can use to meet these needs.

In this sense, the term "resource" applies to both people and things.

Don't worry if it all seems too abstract. In the next pages, many concrete examples will provide you with comprehension and clarity.

Identifying and helping someone experiencing fear

Are you feeling unpleasant sensations in your body? How can you know if they're being caused by fear? Ask yourself these questions:

- Is there someone in my life I would flee from if I could because I believe he, or she, can harm me?

- Is there anyone, or anything else, I believe can do me harm?

- Am I thinking that either I or any of my resources are in danger?

- Will anything happen soon that I believe could harm me?

- Am I about to meet someone who I believe can hurt me or damage some of my resources?

- Is there anyone, or any resource, that I think I'm at risk of losing?

- Am I at risk of losing access to a resource that meets my needs?

If we answer "yes" to any of these similar questions, then it's very likely that we are feeling fear. This doesn't mean fear is the only emotion we are feeling. But it's one of them.

How to deal with fear?

If we can't escape what we believe to be harmful to us, we have at least three options:

1. **Change the odds.** Convince ourselves that what we fear isn't likely to happen.

2. **Create a plan B.** Convince ourselves that even if something bad happens, we'll be ready to deal with it.

3. **Summon allies to deal with the threat.** This involves asking other people for help. This includes talking to anyone we trust and telling them all about the future you. That is, telling them about our fears. These people can help us in many ways. For example, they may help us define a plan B to deal with any bad things that do end up happening. Also, they can help us think more clearly. Are these bad things that likely to happen? Essentially, an ally would help us with options 1 and 2.

How to help someone who is feeling afraid?

We can apply the same suggestions:

- **Help the person to identify** what is *causing* his fear by using the same questions mentioned above.

Become his, or her, ally:

- Help the person **re-evaluate the odds** of something bad happening.

- Help him, or her, create a **plan B.** A strategy that makes this person more self-confident in his, or her, ability to deal with the **situation** he fears or with its **aftermath.**

- Help this person find **more allies.**

The higher the number of sympathetic people coming together to deal with a threat, the smaller the threat will look in the eyes of the person experiencing fear.

Remember that fear, like all the other emotions, exists in degrees. This means that even if we can't eliminate all the fear, we can reduce its degree. At the very least, we can help the person brainstorm ideas to better deal with the threat.

Identifying and calming down someone angry

Are your unpleasant sensations a sign of anger? They could be. Ask yourself the following questions:

- Has anything happened that I consider an injustice?

- Is something going to happen that I think is going to be unjust?

- Is someone doing something to me that I dislike?

- Is anyone, or anything, preventing me from meeting my needs?

- Are there any rules that I believe have been broken?

- Is there any need of mine that is not being met and which I urgently need to meet?

- Are there any boundaries that I think have been crossed by someone else?

- Is there anything in my life that believe I should be trying to change?

Answering "yes" to any of these questions is an indication that anger is one of the emotions triggering the unpleasant feelings you are experiencing.

How to deal with anger?

We feel angry when our brain detects an injustice. Moreover, since our brain focuses on *resources* and *needs*, to deal with anger you have to identify not only the injustice but also **how this injustice relates to our needs and to our resources.** We know we have been successful in this detective work when anger gives way to a new emotion. This emotion is more aligned with the problem in question.

Sounds complicated? Let's look at some examples.

If a person horns at me on the road and I get angry I can ask myself, "What is the need at risk of becoming unfulfilled?" And the answer might be: "The need for peace of mind" or "the need to see people treat each other well." Either way, at the moment I identify these needs, I stop staring at the other person as a threat I need to neutralize as soon as possible. Why? Because my focus has changed.

Before, I was thinking:

- "Who does he think he is?"

- "What? I haven't done anything wrong, why is he honking at me?"

- "I have it when people honk at me"

- "Why are you honking? Can't you see you're the one who almost hit me?"

All these thoughts were ripples from the lightning-fast evaluation my unconscious made of the situation.

That act alone, "someone honking at me when I hadn't done anything wrong," was evaluated as "incorrect, unjust." Furthermore, that single action disturbed my peace of mind and remind me of how inappropriate people sometimes are.

All these evaluations and mental processing happened outside of my conscious awareness. In addition, my brain activated the stress response, transforming my whole body into a war machine. It filled my conscious mind with distressing thoughts about the other person. Then, and only then, did my conscious mind regained control over the situation.

Do you realize how much the world has changed? A few milliseconds ago I was at peace. Then, someone honked at me. And now I'm a different man.

I feel all these stressful changes in my breathing patterns and in my heart rhythm. My head is filled with enemy images. I'm feeling angry.

Fortunately, I knew what to do. I kept asking myself:

- "Why is this situation affecting me so much?"

- "Why is my brain evaluating 'someone honking at me' as a matter of life and death?"

- "What important needs are at stake here?"

And, as my focus shifted so did my underlying rage. Anger gave way to curiosity. Curiosity led me to become my own detective. I kept looking for the needs hidden behind the anger.

By asking myself questions I'm forcing my unconscious mind to become occupied with searching for the answers. Then I realize how much this whole situation affected my peace of mind. I might feel sad for my loss, or I can become afraid: "Am I going to recover the peace I was feeling before?"

Once the needs have been identified, I'm empowered to better deal with the situation. I can ask myself: "How can I act to protect my needs?"

Then, different thoughts will come up in my head. Maybe answers like:

- I can raise my hand and man. Maybe then he'll stop honking and I'll regain my peace of mind.

- I can wait until the traffic flows again, apologize once more just in case and drive away from the man.

- I can distract my mind and make myself think about something else.

- I can count to 10 and take a deep breath.

- I can think of the consequences of acting out my anger. How would that affect my reputation? My family? The relatives of the man who is honking?

- In 20 years, when I remind myself of this situation, what would make me happier: Remembering how I kept my cool while under fire or remembering how I reacted violently to a provocation?

Was anger helpful?

Yes. Anger **alerted** me to how much my world had changed. However, it wasn't helpful in helping me **deal** with the problem.

Sometimes, it's turning anger into another emotion is hard. For example, if my son comes home with a bruised face and I discover that he was beaten by two bullies, how do I feel? I'm enraged. That's normal. After all, what happened was a tremendous injustice!

However, how useful is this anger? The truth is that if I do unto the bullies as they've done to my son, the violence will only continue to escalate, and the consequences will become much worse than a bruised face. People may end up dying. But I can't just stand there and do nothing about it. Fortunately, my degree of angry is so great that it won't let me remain still. It that way, anger is being helpful. But, how to deal with it?

First, I need to identify the needs. These include: (1) The need for my child's well–being, (2) the need to feel safe when my child is at school, (3) the need for justice, and so on.

Then, I ask myself: "How can I act to meet those needs?"

These two steps cause my focus to change. Instead of thinking, "how can I make them pay?" I'm thinking, "How can I meet my needs?"

This helps me think of solutions:

- File a complaint with the school authorities.

- Look for legal counseling about what to do next.

- Consider changing schools.

- Thoroughly analyze my child's school habits to see if he can make some adjustments to his routine that will help him avoid future confrontations.

- Consider talking to the bullies' parents.

- Consider talking to the bullies in the presence of a school authority and the bullies' parents.

- Enroll my child in some type of program that offers specific guidance on how to deal with such problems.

- Seek expert help from a professional trained in helping parents and children cope with such situations.

- Remind myself that many before me have dealt successfully with bullies without ever resorting to violence.

- Ask for help from mature people who have suffered bullying and have been able to solve the problem through peaceful means.

- Read books and articles *online* on the subject.

In this way, my anger will have fulfilled its function It alerted me to the injustice that had occurred and prevented me from ignoring it. Anger motivated me to act. It might even have turned into fear because of the threat hovering over my son. But it's not a paralyzing kind of fear. Rather, it's the type of **fear based on facts that lead me to act** to try to help my child **avoid the outcome** that we both fear.

The point is always the same: when we identify the needs and resources triggering the anger, anger becomes useful. Why? Because it kept us from standing still while witnessing an injustice.

How do you help someone deal with anger?

By empathizing with the important need for justice and by helping the person focus on identifying the needs underlying the anger.

What if anger is being directed against us?

When we suffer from *bullying* or when someone is aggressive it requires a lot of emotional intelligence to get around the situation. Many young people who suffer *bullying* don't know how to deal with this type of psychological violence, which sometimes turns rapidly into physical aggression.

In the case of someone with autism, *bullying* often begins in pre-school, continues in the workplace, and spreads through other social interactions.

Even if someone with autism learns to process emotions to the point of being able to **help** others who are feeling angry, defending **himself** from someone who is *bullying* him is much more complicated.

This is because *bullying* requires an adequate response *at that time.* The autistic person can't go home and meditate on how to defend himself. He can't or to pick up the smartphone and himself how to react.

In this sense, access to simple and easy to understand techniques is essential.

On this subject of dealing with an aggressive person, one of the techniques I like best is the one proposed by Dr. David M. Burns, an adjunct professor emeritus in the Department of Psychiatry and Behavioral Sciences at the Stanford University School of Medicine.

I'm talking about the **disarming technique**. This technique is very easy to memorize and execute. It won't work all the time, especially if we are dealing with someone who just wants to make trouble. However, it's quite helpful when we must deal with criticism and accusations.

In simple terms, when someone calls us names or accuses us of something we have two options to disarm this person:

1. **Calming the person down by finding a way to agree with him.** Whether what the person is saying is right or wrong, try to find a way to find some truth in his remarks. This disarms criticism.

2. **Ask for details.** Ask questions that help the person give you more details about what he dislikes about you. This promotes a healthy dialogue.

When someone is aggressive to us, responding in a like manner just makes things worst. The only way for aggressiveness to work is if we are so aggressive as to make the other person afraid of us. This type of mentality, however, just escalates violence and gives rise to the assaults, hospitalizations, and deaths that fill our news.

On the other hand, finding a way to agree with someone criticizing us or being aggressive, tends to calm the person down. At the same time, asking for examples is a great way to quickly lead the conversation towards a peaceful dialogue. When all is said and done, don't be surprised if the aggressive person ends up apologizing for his attitude.

The key to the technique is that **lying is forbidden**. You can only agree with the person where he is *right.*

What about when you're sure they're wrong? There are two ways you can get around it:

- Agree that *sometimes* you do the things you are being accused of.

- Agree that the person has the right to be angry with *that kind of situation*.

How does this work in practice? Let's look at some examples.

Example 1:

- **Aggressive phrase:** You're worthless!

- **Disarming answer 1:** It's true that I do some things wrong, **(agreeing with the aggressor)**, are you thinking of anything specific? **(Asking for details).**

- **Disarming answer 2:** I understand that you are very disturbed by something that happened **(agreeing that the person is angry)** can you tell me what happened? **(Asking for details).**

Example 2:

- **Aggressive phrase:** Why don't you ever do anything right?

- **Disarming answer 1:** I see I did something that you'd like me to have done differently **(agreeing)**, can you tell me what it was? **(Asking for details)**

- **Disarming answer 2:** I see that you like things to be done right **(agreeing)** can you tell me what I did wrong? **(Asking for details).**

- **Disarming answer 3:** I can understand, it's frustrating when we want something done right and we see others aren't helping **(agreeing that it is normal for this kind of situation to be disturbing to a person)** can you tell me where I could have been of more help to you? **(Asking for details).**

Example 3:

- **Aggressive phrase:** You are the dumbest student this school has ever had!

- **Disarming answer 1:** Yeah, sometimes I don't really understand things, **(agreeing)**, can you tell me what you would like me to understand better? **(Asking for details while recognizing that, no matter how much you understand something, you can always get better).**

- **Disarming answer 2:** It must be frustrating when you really want me to learn something and you see that I can't **(agreeing)**, among the things that you've tried to teach me before, which one are you thinking about? **(Asking for details).**

- **Disarming answer 3 if the accusation is false:** It must be discouraging when a student doesn't learn at the pace the teacher wants **(agreeing with the general principle: "It's discouraging for any teacher when a student fails to learn as fast as the teacher wants")**, what do you wish me to understand better? **(Asking for details, giving the person an opportunity to reveal what he is thinking about).**

Example 4:

- **Aggressive phrase:** You will never be anyone in your life.

- **Disarming answer 1:** That's a possibility. I too, dislike it. **(agreeing with the general principle but without agreeing with the aggressive person's prediction)**, can you tell me where I could improve? **(Asking for details in a non-threatening way).**

- **Disarming answer 2:** I can see this is worrying you a lot **(agreeing that the person is worried)**, can you explain me better why do you believe that? **(Asking for details).**

In each case, the aggressive phrase came from someone in battle mode. Words became arrows in his mouth, trying to pierce you and win the war.

However, your non-contradictory reaction sends a clear message to that person's limbic system:

- You are not a threat.

This makes it easier for a more pleasant dialogue to develop.

In addition to the disarming technique, there is another effective method, "the Benjamin Franklin effect."

The Benjamin Franklin effect

Benjamin Franklin was one of the founding fathers of the United States and is recognized as the inventor of the lightning rod.

In his autobiography, he described how he dealt with the rivalry of a political adversary:

> « Having heard that he had in his library a certain very scarce and curious book, I wrote a note to him, expressing my desire of perusing that book, and requesting he would do me the favor of lending it to me for a few days. He said it immediately, in I returned it in about a week with another note, expressing strongly my sense of the favor. When we next met in the House [of Representatives], he spoke to me (which he had never done before), and with great civility; and he ever after manifested a readiness to serve me on all occasions, so that we become great friends, and our friendship continued to his death. »[4]

Why would ask for a small favor work so well? As it turns out, our brain likes to be congruent. It's as if the unconscious part of our brain reasoned: "I don't like that person, but I did him a favor. How could I have done him a favor if I didn't like him? Obviously,

---

[4]Link: http://www.ushistory.org/franklin/autobiography/page48.htm

I must like him a little bit. Yes, that makes *more sense* than to believe that I don't like him."

This process is described in psychology as our brain's need to solve the so-called cognitive dissonances — differences in thinking.

This is the reason why we tend to enjoy a product more *right after* we've bought it. Again, it is as if the unconscious part of our brain is thinking, "Well, I was uncertain as to whether this product was good or not, but I did buy it, didn't I? Surely, this means I'm wasn't as uncertain as I thought."

All of this makes sense. But, there might be another reason.

For example, have you noticed how people get all excited and happy when you ask them for directions? Try it out. Next time you are out on the street, ask for directions to the nearest supermarket. You'll probably marvel at people reactions.

What's going on?

As we have already noted, contributing to the wellbeing of others is one of the fundamental needs we have. Someone who is critical or aggressive may not even have noticed it, but the truth is that when he does something that contributes to the well-being of another person, he feels satisfied.

There is just something you need to keep in mind. When a favor is too big and requires a lot of physical or mental energy, it may end up causing some degree of disgust.

However, when it comes to small favors, this may result in a feeling of satisfaction. You've just made the aggressive person associate "feeling good" with "doing good to you."

How can you apply these principles and gain the favor of someone aggressive?

Ask for little favors. Simple things. Then, express your sincere gratitude. True, it may be difficult to know where to start. Here are some examples to help you out:

- Can you tell me what time is it? Thank you very much.

- What's our next class? Thank you so much for your help.

- Can you pass me that, please? Thank you. I appreciate that.

- Can you hold on to this for a moment? That was so kind of you. Thank you so much.

You can also ask for some advice or opinion:

- Hi! I know you're a great player of [name of the game]. Can you help me figure out how to beat this level?

- I'm torn between these two options; can you help me decide which one I should choose?

The process is always the same: ask for something that the person has satisfaction in doing for you. Something simple, that won't cause disgust.

Of course, some bullies at school can be quite resilient, but perseverance in being kind will certainly bring good results.

Identifying and helping someone experience Disgust

What questions can help you determine if the unpleasant sensations you are feeling area a sign of disgust?

- Do I feel nauseous?

- Do I feel like vomiting?

- Am I about to do something I wish I wouldn't have to do?

- Am I going to meet someone who wastes my mental energy?

- Have I just been with something or someone who has wasted either my mental or physical energy?

- Was I forced to stop doing something I was enjoying?

- Is there anything in my life that I wish wasn't part of it?

- Am I feeling mentally tired?

- Is my brain rejecting everything? Even thinking?

Disgust is difficult to identify and often goes unnoticed. But, because it's intimately connected with the mental and physical energy we have available, there's a simple rule you can follow if you have autism: If you are mentally tired and have to interact with someone, you'll be feeling *disgust*.

How should you deal with disgust?

The best way to deal with disgust is twofold. If you're fatigued, you need to rest your mind. You need to be quiet, lying down, maybe listening to some relaxing music.

However, sometimes, being physically at rest doesn't mean your mind will be recovering. Why?

Well, suppose you are feeling nauseous (a sign of disgust) at the thought of having to deal with a troublesome person tomorrow. In this case, standing still won't be of help because your mind will have the tendency to keep ruminating on the subject — wasting your remaining mental stamina. This means it may be necessary to get involved in some activity that you really enjoy. When you have autism this often involves isolating yourself with a favorite pastime — oftentimes referred to as an "obsession" for lack of a better term to describe the degree of fascination someone with autism can develop for a topic of interest.

Tony Attwood, considered the world's leading Asperger's syndrome specialist, recommends that for every hour spent in the company of people, someone with Asperger should spend an hour alone, resting his mind. Later in this book, we will talk more about the wear and tear that people cause on someone with autism.

For now, just keep in mind that just as *anger* is a strong emotion that *leads us closer* to the situation and *moves us to act*, disgust leads us to *reject the situation* and *motivates us to move away from it*.

In addition, we can try to identify what needs or resources are at stake, underlying disgust. In most cases, the need being disturbed is the need to rest your head. However, if getting away and resting doesn't attenuate disgust, this is a sign that there are other needs involved.

How to help someone who is experiencing disgust?

It's essential to help the person to move away from the stimulus causing the reaction. Forcing the person to continue to process this stimulus, or to continue to interact with the person who is triggering disgust, is a bad idea. Why? Because it will cause disgust to increase to the point of repugnance. Moreover, forcing an autistic person to interact when he is already tired may lead to a strong nervous breakdown — a *meltdown.*

Identifying and helping someone Surprised

Surprise usually lasts only for a few moments. When it lasts longer than that, we refer to it as "shock" and often say that we are shocked and that we have not yet processed, or assimilated, what happened.

So, what questions help us see if the unpleasant sensations we are feeling evidence surprise?

- Did something happen that was different than of what I was expecting?

- Did something happen that shocked me?

- Did something happen that confused me?

How to handle surprise?

Once again, the solution is to take the time to process everything. In addition, the help of an understanding friend who is familiar with autism will be of great help.

How to help someone who is feeling shocked or confused?

Feelings of surprise signal the need to process new and unexpected information. Some well-placed questions will help the surprised person do this. These include:

- What happened?

- Why did that surprise you?

- What were you expecting to happen?

- Why do you think things happened differently?

- How do you think things will change in the future because of what happened?

- What are the negative aspects of what happened?

- What are the good points?

- How can you adapt to deal with the negative aspects?

- Who can I help you?

- What can I do for you right now to help you deal with this situation?

We want to help the person build a narrative. This narrative includes the answer to these questions:

- Why did this happen?

- How did it change things?

- What do I need to do to adapt to what happened?

When the person understands this, he will be ready to overcome the shock. But that isn't the end of the story. Now, depending on your new understanding of the future, you may be afraid, disgusted, angry, or sad, and you will have to deal with these new emotions accordingly.

Identifying and helping someone feeling sad.

Are you feeling sad? Ask yourself these questions:

- Did I lose something, someone or a pet?

- Is someone I love, or a pet, sick?

- Has anyone I love died?

- Has anyone I love moved away?

- Is there someone I wish was here with me but who is not?

- Did something happen that made me lose my self-respect or my desire to live?

- Have I been diagnosed with a health problem?

- Am I thinking that something bad is going to happen to something or someone I love?

All these questions have a common theme: loss. Whether it's real or imagined, the idea of losing something or someone precious to us causes sadness.

How to deal with sadness and help others?

Sadness will lessen when at least two goals are achieved:

1. **We give our mind enough time to rearrange its thought processes.**

   In the case of a large loss, such as the death of a loved one, this can take a long time.

2. **We find a new resource or a new strategy to meet the needs that were once met by that which was lost.**

And to accelerate the process of achieving both goals, we can ask two types of questions:

1. **Questions aimed at helping others explain why what was lost was so important.**

   These kinds of questions are the ones that help the person to establish a relationship between the lost resource and his own needs.

2. **Questions that help them reason about how to adjust their life to find new resources to meet those needs.**

These kinds of questions help the person understand how to use other resources to meet those same needs.

Let's look at some practical examples. And of course, bear in mind that such questions should be asked *only* when the person is prepared. Depending on the magnitude of the loss, you may have to wait several days, or even weeks, until the person becomes capable of reasoning about what has been lost.

- Questions aimed at helping others explain why what was lost was so important.

    o Why did you like this person?

    o What did you enjoy most about his personality?

    o How did this person help you?

    o What did you do for him?

    o In what ways do you think you depended on him?

    o How did your life change now that this person is gone?

    o Why did you like your pet?

    o What did you use to do together?

    o What do you miss the most?

    o How has your life changed now that it is gone?

    o Why was this object so important to you?

    o What did you use it for?

- How did your life change now that you've lost it?

For example, if someone has lost a brother he has lost more than just "one person." He suffered the loss of a friend, a confidant, and a playmate. It may be necessary to find several people to take on each of these roles.

It's not about replacing the lost person. It's just that even after such a great loss you continue to need friends, confidants, and playmates.

When we suffer a loss, we increase our chances of coping with it by finding new ways to meet our needs. No one can replace the lost person, but many people may try to satisfy the same needs as this person once did, even if to a lesser extent. This will lessen the feeling of despair.

- Questions that can help someone to find new resources to meet his needs:

    - What other valuable people do you have in your life?

    - What kind of help do they need?

    - What can you do to help one of them tomorrow?

    - How will helping them satisfy your need to contribute to the wellbeing of others?

    - How do these people contribute to your wellbeing?

    - What is your favorite animal that you would like to have as a pet?

    - Why?

    - Do you think that one day you will be ready to take care of another pet?

- What do you think about going to one of your friend's house to play with his pet?

- What other objects can you use to achieve the same goal as the lost object?

- If the lost object had been gifted by a loved one and was a memory, you could ask: "What other objects do you have that help you remember that person?"

Reverse Engineering Emotions

In this chapter, we got a concrete understanding of emotions and their role in our life. This concrete understanding allows us to reverse engineer emotions. How?

If the someone with autism is feeling angry and doesn't know *why*, he can use the questions outlined earlier in this chapter to unearth the injustice his brain has detected.

All these questions help the autistic person to do *manually* what his brain should have done *automatically.* The good news is that due to the neuroplastic characteristics of our brain, over time, this manual process will become increasingly automatized.

With training, the person with autism will process things faster and faster. For example, after going through this process several times, you may notice there are 2 or 3 needs that arise most often.

"I suffered an injustice! This means my need for *respect* wasn't taken into consideration. This makes me angry. But if I've *lost* respect this loss also makes me feel sad. What can I do to deal with this situation without being aggressive?"

And, what would have taken many minutes, or hours, to process, is now being dealt with in a few moments.

Of course, all of this presupposes that the person with autism has a more moderate form of this condition, such as Asperger's syndrome.

Someone with a deeper form of autism, where even basic communication is affected, will have a harder time grasping these abstract concepts. It may take him many years. But for those on the spectrum who can read, even reading this chapter may be enough to change the way they deal with the strange sensations arising in their body, the emotions. This understanding may become life-changing.

Still on the topic of emotions, surely you have noticed the autistic tendency to flap their limbs and hands, rock on a chair or make noises with their mouth. What's at the root of these behaviors? How should a parent interpret them? In the next chapter, we'll dive into this topic.

Chapter 5

Unraveling the Mysteries of Stimming

I magine you're talking to someone about your favorite topic. You are very enthusiastic, but you notice how the other person keeps tapping his foot. You ignore this. "I'm almost done with my explanation," you reason. However, the more you explain, the more fantastic ideas come to mind.

The minutes pass and you don't even notice. Only your voice is heard. The other person no longer looks at you, he just stares at his watch wondering when the conversation will end. His hands don't stop either. He crosses his arms for a moment, only to move his hands to his hips, trouser pockets, and back to the hips again.

Well, there's no doubt your listener is impatient. But what we want to know is: **Why do people move their limbs when they get impatient?**

This happens for at least two reasons. First, it's a polite way of showing the other person he needs to end the conversation. Secondly, these movements calm us down.

It's a fact that movement exerts a calming effect. The more the better. Several clinical studies show the calming and antidepressant properties of physical exercise. Anyone of us who has ever come home physically exhausted after a day's work knows that feeling of just wanting to get to bed and rest.

Parents see this in their children too. When they spend the day outside, running and playing with the ball, they get tired and calmer.

Want to try this out? Go for a walk whenever you are anxious. The movement will calm you down.

With this in mind, let's recall one of the basic characteristics of autism: When someone has autism, the areas responsible for modeling emotions don't work correctly. In practice, this means it's difficult for the autistic person to control the intensity of what they are feeling.

A few pages back we saw the effect this has on how a young autistic boy dealt with his emotions in comparison with a neurotypical boy.

A young neurotypical instinctively feels the need to vent, to distract himself with an activity, or to think about other things.

Conversely, a young autist uses a different strategy to reduce the intensity of his emotions. He flaps his hands, jumps, dances, rocks himself back and forth in a chair, moves erratically, pulls his hair, scribbles a sheet of paper, makes noises with his mouth, claps, rolls over on the floor or onto a bed, rubs interesting textures, and so on.

Whatever works to reduce somewhat the intensity of the unpleasant sensations caused by the emotions he has so much difficulty in understanding and controlling.

These movements are known by an English expression called *stimming*.

But not all the stimming is good. Some strategies of stimming are bad, such as: hurting himself or someone else, overthrowing things, acting violently, yelling at others. So, what to do?

You need to prevent your child from hurting himself or other people, but how can you do this in a way that allows your child to continue to have a way to calm down?

How to deal with the stimming of someone with moderate autism, such as Asperger's syndrome?

As a parent, watching your child flapping his hands can be shocking. It's understandable if you feel the need to stop the child. But doing so would be a terrible idea. Why?

Because stimming is how someone with autism handles nervous tension and the intensity of his emotions. We all have this need to control the unpleasant sensations in our body. In the case of the autistic, stimming is the strategy of choice to satisfy this need.

Because of this, preventing stimming causes the person to develop nervous tics, tremors — on the lips and the eyelids, for example — and leads to nervous breakdowns. Prohibiting stimming is also a guarantee that the autistic person will eventually fall into depression.

It may be hard to hear this. But there's nothing one can do. Stimming is a part of autism just as breathing is a part of being human.

So how do you act if your child exhibits destructive stimming?

It's necessary to encourage the child to replace the destructive stimming with a harmless alternative. Show the child how to stim. Maybe other parents will think you are crazy for teaching your child all about the benefits of rolling in bed or flapping his hands.

But it's your son.

His brain doesn't have the neurological connections needed to regulate the intensity of his emotions. If you don't teach him how to stim the right way, who will? It'll be a matter of time until the destructive stimming causes problems and brings suffering to your whole family.

As soon as you can, teach your child about the need to do stim in a smart way. Teach him that when he is in a public place, and all those nasty sensations arise, making him want to run away or scream, it's essential to get into a public restroom or to look for another reserved place and flap his hands or jump until he calms himself down.

Once he's old enough to understand, explain to him what emotions are, using a concrete teaching style. Use as many examples as needed. Use videos, pictures, and drawings to illustrate your points. Adapt these examples to the age and degree of autism of the child, adolescent or adult.

Whenever possible, use examples related to his special interests. If he loves trains use this theme as the basis for your examples. If he loves Star Wars use that. Do this and you will change the life of your child forever.

Once your child gains a greater understanding of the unpleasant sensations he feels, you can help him find even better ways to calm down. These include staying alone in a quiet place while he engages in a favorite activity, such as listening to music or art creation.

How to deal with stimming when it comes from someone with a deeper form of autism?

If your child has a deeper form of autism, teaching him the basics of emotional intelligence can be next to impossible. What should you do?

The most effective way to connect with someone with deep autism might be mimicking their stimming.

If your child is wobbling on the floor, lie on the floor and wobble with him. If he is flapping his hands, flap your hands with him.

It sounds crazy. But just try it.

I wouldn't believe it works if I hadn't tried it myself. It's, perhaps, the most effective way to connect with the profoundly autistic, regardless of the age or degree of autism.

Over time, you may enter your child's inner world and gain a greater capacity to influence his behavior.

Moreover, if your child can't talk, it's vital that you interpret his stimming as a form of communication. But what's the child trying to communicate?

The important message behind stimming

When someone stims, interpret that as if the person was shaking.

If a child is shaking, no loving father says, "Stop that!" Quite the contrary. The father gets the message: His son is freezing. So, he'll try to get him warmer clothes or a blanket.

However, if the tremors continue, this father understands something more serious is triggering this symptom. Is the child afraid of something? Does he have a fever? Is he having some type of seizure and is in need of immediate medical attention?

A loving father is like that. He is aware of the signs his son gives him, especially when that son is a baby and can't communicate. Every cry is met with attention and curiosity: "Is the baby hungry? Uncomfortable? In pain? Why? How can I help him?"

In the same way, the father of someone with autism needs to construe stimming as a communication tool.

Stimming is how the autistic lets you know something isn't right with him.

The deeper the autism, the greater the difficulty of the autistic person in communicating what is happening to him. In that sense, the deep autistic is like a baby. Why?

Because a baby who is shaking is dependent on the father to realize he needs a blanket. In the same way, a person with a deep level of autism depends on the ability of his parents to identify what's creating in him the need to stim.

In the previous chapter we looked at a common source: emotions. Strong emotions cause feelings. Stimming helps the autistic person deal with them and reduce their intensity.

This applies even with a pleasant sensation. For example, if someone tickles you, you giggle. But if you continue to be tickled that pleasurable feeling quickly becomes intolerable. The same thing happens in autism. That's why the autistic stims even when he feels happy.

He jumps, screams, and wobbles with happiness. It's just his brain trying to exert control over the intensity of his feelings. Since his brain can't control emotions through the normal pathways, it uses external means such as body movements.

In fact, your autistic child is a genius. From an early age, he discovered that through stimming he was able to modulate the intensity of his sensations. He is like a hacker who, upon losing his email account password, still found a way to get into his account and read his emails.

But emotions aren't the only causes of stimming.

In the next chapter, we will look at another common source of unpleasant sensations that lead to stimming: sensory stimuli.

Chapter 6

Sensory Hypersensitivity — A Fundamental Aspect of the Autistic Brain Frequently Ignored

While a baby cries to signal a need or an unpleasant or sensation, such as a bellyache., the autistic stims.

But physical sensations are just one kind of sensory stimuli our brain can process.

The human brain processes information relating to various senses. How many? We usually think of five:

- Sight.

- Hearing.

- Touch.

- Smell.

- Taste.

However, we now know there are many other senses. These include, for example:

- The senses coordinated by the vestibular system present in our ears. This system handles our ability to perceive the **direction, acceleration,** and **inclination** of our body. This allows us to keep our **balance** and to **adjust our posture.**

- **Thermoception** — the ability to feel temperature. Generally, when we talk about the sense of touch, we end up including the ability to feel temperature, although it is a separate sense.

- **Proprioception** — also called the kinesthetic sense. That is, the perception of the location of our own limbs (arms and legs) in space. That's how our body knows where each limb is, relative to the others and how the strength each muscle is exerting. It is the ability of proprioception that allows us to touch our nose even when our eyes are closed, and it's this sense that gives a well-trained athlete the ability to drive the ball with his feet even when his eyes are fixed on the goal.

- **Nociception** — the perception of pain. Again, this is another sense often confused with touch. Even though we have pressure sensors responsible for the sense of touch, there are three other types of receptors responsible for the perception of pain. These allow us to receive pain signals from (1) our skin, (2) our bones and joints, and (3) our internal organs.

Besides these, our body also has sensors involved in detecting the level of salt in our blood. That way, our brain keeps being notified about salt levels in our blood. If these rise too much, we feel thirsty.

Likewise, many other sensors relate to other sensations, such as hunger. These senses are intimately connected with our needs, as we have already seen.

In addition, each of these senses can be divided into smaller aspects.

The sense of sight, to illustrate, involves the processing of colors, textures, shapes, three-dimensional perspective, lines, and the relationship between these and the light waves reaching the objects in front of us, as they move and change location.

Also, hearing involves volume, rhythm, tone, the processing of any information present in the sounds we hear, such as words or music, and the separation of these sounds from the background noise. Oftentimes, we don't think about the extraordinary processing machine that is our brain. A real supercomputer.

All this processing depends on specialized neural networks, the areas or modules, responsible for digesting the information and conveying its conclusions to the other areas. In this way, the whole brain works together to build an inner model of the real world. A rich sensory experience.

Autism and sensory perception

Let's take a closer look at each of the senses we've described. In autism, there are three possibilities for each of them. They are:

1. Hypersensitivity.

2. Normal sensitivity.

3. Hyposensitivity.

We'll begin by analyzing a sense in which each of these three characteristics is easy to understand. Then we will explore the remaining sensory channels.

Hearing

We all like music and we all have a favorite volume to listen to it. Some of us like it loud, others prefer a quieter soundscape.

Besides, we all have different genre preferences. While some of us enjoy the low-frequency beats present in many popular songs, others favor the classical compositions with their instrumental richness and varied rhythms.

This diversity is normal, it's part of what makes us unique.

However, this uniqueness can be quite pronounced in someone with autism.

How would you feel if you had to work with a pneumatic hammer without wearing an earmuff? The noise would cause you great discomfort and you could even end up with an earache.

We this example in mind, we can see that we all have a volume limit. Some of us can stand in front of powerful booming speakers and enjoy it, while others would get annoyed, even disgusted, with the experience.

Something similar happens in autism. It's just that this volume tolerance can be much lower. It's not uncommon to find individuals who not only dislike a certain sound but can't stand them. These unbearable sounds cause them discomfort, even pain. However, most people without autism would consider these sounds enjoyable.

If you have an autistic child, note how he reacts as you increase the volume of the music you are listening to. Did he cover his ears when the music was still in a volume you consider acceptable? If he did, then this means that, for his brain, the music sounded like a pneumatic hammer.

If your child has Asperger's syndrome or another form of moderate autism, a slightly louder song may make him verbalize his discomfort: "Turn down the music! It's too loud!" But in the case of a child with deep autism, the only visible sign that something isn't right will be the stimming behavior.

This means that your child can be on a good, quiet day, and suddenly, as you turn on the radio, he starts screaming, rolling on the floor or even crying. What is going on?

It just so happens that the volume you chose, while perfectly acceptable to you, sounds like an airplane taking off inside his head. Since he can't verbalize his discomfort, much less modulate the disgust he is feeling, he reacts through stimming.

This stimming fulfilled two functions: it calmed him down a little, and it signaled you to lower the volume. It's as if his stimming said: "Turn off the speakers! My ears are killing me!" Many times, however, those around fail to grasp the message hidden within the stimming.

In addition, the very frequency of sounds can be a problem. Low-frequency beats, like those produced by a subwoofer, can be a source of torment. The same is true for high-pitched tunes. This means a motorbike, a siren, or an alarm, can trigger a state of emergency within the autistic brain.

If you want to find out who has autism, wait for an ambulance to pass by, with its sirens honking, and watch who covers their ears and writhes in pain. These are the people with sound hypersensitivity and there is a good chance they'll have some degree of autism.

Although less common, the opposite is also possible. The autistic brain may be hyposensitive to some frequencies or sounds. This can make language interpretation difficult, causing the person to struggle to understand certain syllables.

As if all this weren't enough, in the case of deep autism, sound can be processed in such a divergent way that it becomes impossible for the autistic person to have an adequate perception of what is real.

Can you remember what happens when you are asleep and dreaming and the noises outside are affecting what you see and hear in the dream? Based on existing accounts that might be how the outer world sounds like to someone profoundly affected by autism.

A great example is that of Tito Rajarshi Mukhopadhyay, mentioned by Temple Grandin. He is the author of *Beyond the Silence: My Life, the World and Autism*. Although his brain is set up in a way that prevents him from activating his vocal chords and talking, he has learned to read and write on his computer. His writings gave us a window into the world of the deeply autistic, which differs greatly from what the researchers believed!

And that goes to show the potential of the human brain for learning and **communication**, even for someone who has deep autism.

Sight

Visual hypersensitivity is nothing like sound hypersensitivity. Why?

Because anyone can distinguish between a low and a high volume even if they don't have sound hypersensitivity.

This can make life easier for you. As you get to know the particularities of your child's autism you'll get better at discerning what sounds the child can, and cannot, tolerate.

Unfortunately, with visual hypersensitivity, things aren't this linear.

Did you know some lights flicker? For example, fluorescent lights can get distracting, even disturbing, to someone on the spectrum, rather quickly. They may be at the root of headaches, stimming and nervous breakdowns.

In addition, the autistic brain can become overwhelmed with visual information. How does this happen?

Imagine that you are in a supermarket, looking for a specific brand of juice. As your eyes roam the shelves you are faced with dozens of labels trying to capture your attention. One by one, your brain processes them all, comparing the name in the label with the one you are looking for.

You don't even notice it but, in the space of a few minutes, your visual system processes innumerable visual details. All this, at the expense of some mental energy. However, because everything is set up properly inside your skull, you don't see it happening.

Things can be very different for someone with autism.

As a rule, someone with autism has many difficulties in ignoring sensory stimuli.

As someone with moderate autism - Asperger's Syndrome - expressed himself:

> « As I am driving my car, my brain is not just processing information about the other cars. I'm paying attention to the surrounding buildings, to the details on the road, to the noise of the wind, to the temperature of my body, to the bench I'm sitting on and the pressure it makes on my body. All at the same time. It is as if my brain cannot isolate and ignore sensory stimuli. This is especially annoying when I want to sleep or when I want to focus on a task. Anything distracts me. Hence, I prefer to listen

to music loud enough to isolate the other noises and distractions. But it must be music I already know well, otherwise, those new lyrics and rhythms become distracting. »

Due to this impotence to ignore sensory stimuli, how does someone with autism feel when faced with a lot of visual information?

Well, imagine that there are 50 people around you. They are all speaking at the same time about different topics. Usually, you would try to pay attention to just one of them. But what if you couldn't ignore any of them?

You try to pay attention and respond to each of them but you can't. Your head gets tired. You no longer feel like processing whatever they're saying. You only hope to get out of there.

That's why your autistic child gets impatient in shopping malls. It's like all those colorful labels are trying to grab his attention, wasting his precious mental stamina.

The same is true for other places containing many visual and auditory details. All this sensory input will end up in an endless brain queue. This excess of information will cause disgust, nausea and even a kind of nervous breakdown we will discuss in the next chapter.

In addition, visual hypersensitivity may manifest itself as a strong intolerance to light. Just as loud sounds may cause ear pain, a strong light can cause a headache and ocular distress.

Besides shopping malls, supermarkets and any other places with lots of information to process, simpler things can also become as distressing as having to attend to 50 different people at the same time. But what kind of "simpler" things are we talking about? Complex patterns and bright colors.

It's true. Clothing with checkered patterns of various colors, shapes, or motifs, may be all that is needed to bring an autistic brain to its knees.

You put on your favorite blouse and your autistic child starts stimming. You do not even notice the relationship, but it's there.

Now imagine: suppose your home, including your child's room, is decorated with lots of colorful ornaments, plus a wallpaper with a pattern and curtains with intense colors. If your child has visual hypersensitivity, being at home will be a sensory nightmare.

For your child, being at home is like being between two supermarket shelves: exhausting and repulsive. However, from the point of view of any other neurotypical person, your home is an example of decorum and good taste. who would have guessed?

In addition to visual hypersensitivity, hyposensitivity also exists. The latter manifests itself through a difficulty in being stimulated by visual information. A kind of blindness where the eyes see but the brain doesn't process it right away. A child with this kind of sensory processing disorder may not react to a new visual stimulus unless it is sufficiently different and compelling.

For example, the child may not detect, or react, to a dimmer light source. Likewise, he may get easily distracted, as his eyes fail to recognize where they should be focusing.

For all the other children, it's obvious that the chalkboard is the main element in the room. However, to the visual hyposensitive child, the higher stimulation coming from the window, with its glowing sunrays, may be much more appealing.

Hyper and hyposensitive in any of the senses are dependent on how the areas of the brain responsible for sensory processing were affected during brain development.

Smell

Someone with autism can develop sensitivities to many different smells. Some may refer to these hypersensitivities as "allergies" because they don't know the appropriate term to describe their experience. But one thing they know: strong smells affect them — a lot!

Again, the opposite may also be true: hyposensitivity to some smells and an attraction to those kinds of smells most people find quite unpleasant, such as the smell of your own sweat.

Based on my observation, odors of artificial origin cause more hypersensitivity problems than natural aromas, even if that natural smell is unpleasant.

Every autistic person is different, and you need to be aware of what affects your child — or yourself — and do what you can to avoid prolonged contact with these scents.

Touch and nociception — the perception of pain

Touch is one of the senses where the dichotomy between "hypersensitivity and hyposensitivity" is more pronounced.

On the one hand, being touch by other people can be quite unpleasant.

Not infrequently, the autistic person will avoid being touched. This includes avoiding hugs, handshakes, and kisses. So, don't be surprised if your child cleans his face right after being kissed by auntie — or, from his perspective, being licked by a slimy, cold and viscous liquid. That's right, a child with autism can feel about kisses on the cheek in the same way a neurotypical person feels about being licked vigorously by a drooling dog.

In fact, it is not uncommon to hear someone with a moderate form of autism say, "I don't like being touched." Why does this happen? Again, the answer lies in how the various neural networks involved in the processing of touch process this sensory information.

Do you know those people that keep hitting you with their hand while they talk to you? Sometimes they engage in this kind of behavior to guarantee you keep looking at them, or to emphasize their point. For an autistic person with touch hypersensitivity, this would feel like being jab by the tip of a broom. Quite uncomfortable, don't you agree?

At the same time, it is easy to hurt a hypersensitive person, as nociception receptors can be much more sensitive. A handshake that the neurotypical feels firm can be a painful finger-crushing grab. A "pat" on the back is perceived as a violent blow to the back.

Another complex subject, responsible for much suffering, is clothing. Skin-rubbing labels and scratching fibers can lead the autistic brain to madness.

Parents of autistic children sometimes complain that their children persist in undressing their clothes. This is a clear indication you need to buy clothing with softer fibers.

In fact, this field is yet another way to find out who is on the autistic spectrum. Notice who wears the same clothing every time. Not necessarily the same piece, but the same set of 3 or 4 pieces. These have in common their soft fibers and colors.

Moreover, worn-out clothing is smoother, so the autistic person can end up wearing the same clothes for years, even if these clothes are already old and outdated. Another common aspect involves the tendency to wear clothing a size, or more, above. Again, the extra comfort provided is the reason for this choice.

A young man who worked at an IT company complained to me about a co-worker who wore the same t-shirt every day, didn't bathe and had a terrible smell of sweat.

Well, do you see here a probable Asperger's? Notice: The same clothing, hyposensitivity to the smell of his own sweat and a dislike for bathing Wait! What's the connection between bath aversion and autism?

Why the bath aversion?

Bathing means going through temperature changes. It breaks your routine. You need to change clothes. And you know that feeling you get on your skin after spreading the soap? That can be a problem too.

Not all autistics have an aversion to bathing though. After all, bathing can be quite pleasant and relaxing, but aversion can happen and you'd better be prepared for it.

If your child hates to bathe try, for example, preheating the bathroom so that the temperature change is less pronounced.

However, while we have someone with an aversion to being touched — and completing what we said before about the dichotomy of touch — we also have someone who loves to feel pressure on his body.

He doesn't like hugs. True. Unless the hug is tight. It's normal to see autistic people squeezing themselves into tight spaces or sleeping under many blankets. Why? Because the pressure soothes the autistic brain — it's a form of stimming.

This's doesn't mean you should squeeze your child. It's important to let him choose when and for how long he wants to be squeezed. Otherwise, you may end up disturbing him even more.

Besides pressure, other pleasant forms of stimulation involving touch used by autistic people include caressing rough textures with their skin or lips, rubbing pebbles between their fingers, and shoving their hands in baskets of dried beans.

Taste

Have you ever watched your child removing each pea from his plate before eating? Refusing to eat fish? Grouping potatoes, meat, and vegetables eating them separately? Demanding to eat the same food every day?

These are some of the consequences of taste hypersensitivity.

To reduce his sensory discomfort, your child can go to great lengths to ensure that not a single pea, or any other flavor he's sensitive to, ends up inside his mouth.

Fishbones, for example, can cause such an unpleasant sensation in his mouth that he can refuse eating fish altogether.

Also, although he enjoys the taste of potatoes and loves the texture of the meat, the two together don't work in his mouth —

at least not at the same time. What's the simplest solution? Eat them separately. Problem solved.

And what about that steak with rice you made yesterday? It's so difficult to find a meal containing the perfect balance of textures and flavors and do you want to know something? Your white rice with grilled steak is the epitome of perfection for your child's taste buds. So, could you prepare this meal for lunch and dinner, every day, for the rest of your life?

On the other hand, forcing him to eat something he doesn't want causes stimming and may even lead to a nervous breakdown.

What can you do?

When your child refuses to eat, your first step involves making a very important distinction: Is he throwing a tantrum or is it hypersensitivity?

It's difficult to know the answer if your child can't communicate it to you. You need to do some detective work. If your child has eaten that food in the past and liked it and if now he's stimming when you try to give it to him, it's probably a tantrum. But if he always refuses to eat that particular food, hypersensitivity might be at play here.

Does this mean your child will never eat fish or peas?

No. But it means you must find a way to make these foods more appealing to him. This may involve using spices or other seasonings to modify both the taste and the smell of the food. You can also try different cooking methods and play around with the texture and appearance of the meal.

Use your imagination and keep adjusting each variable. Can you grind the fish and mix it with another food he enjoys? There are several ways to deal with the problem of food rejection and over time you will adapt your cooking habits to your child's hypersensitivities.

And what about hyposensitivity? This isn't too problematic. Maybe your child loves boiling hot food and refuses to eat the food after it has warmed. Maybe he has an unusual drive for salty or spicy food.

These differences in taste are part of being human, whether we are autistic or neurotypical. But in autism, due to difficulties in modeling the intensity of emotions, a hypersensitivity may end up becoming another reason for much stimming or a nerve crisis.

As an example, many people without autism prefer salty food over a sweet treat, but they won't have a nervous breakdown because there's only cake for dessert. Hence the need to know your child's peculiarities. This will allow you to predict nervous breakdown and prepare for it.

The vestibular system and proprioception

Motor coordination can be a challenge for someone with autism. Why? Because the neural networks responsible for pinpointing the position of the limbs may not be communicating this location to the areas coordinating muscular contraction and movement. It's like attempting to follow the directions of a GPS that keeps second-guessing itself. The result may be a person who has a very unusual gait, or a young man who simply doesn't fit on the soccer team.

After all, imagine driving a car with a loose steering wheel and a speedometer displaying the wrong speed. Anyone who is observing the jerky motions of the car would think you are a bad driver, when in fact, the car is the issue. Likewise, if your autistic child is clumsy, the problem lays in the inner workings of his brain. It's not something he can directly control.

This doesn't mean he can't improve with proper training or that he can't become very good at some type of sport or activity, but it means it'll be harder for him.

To illustrate, our fingers are much more tailored to playing the piano than our toes. Coordinating the movement of each individual toe with precision is troublesome for our brain. However, videos of people playing piano with their feet are not uncommon. This exemplifies the challenges training and perseverance can overcome.

Our brain is plastic. It adapts. Someone with autism simply starts with a disadvantage.

However, under normal circumstances, don't be surprised if your child occasionally misses the door and ends up hitting the door frame or if he ends up hurting you with his teeth while trying to kiss you. The truth is that for him, the simple act of slowing down his face just enough so it gently collides with your cheek can be as complicated as landing the lunar module intact on the surface of the moon.

Moreover, performing seemingly simple tasks such as tying his shoes can be a challenge. This is because the areas related to precise movements, such as those performed by the fingers, tend to be among the underdeveloped areas in the autistic brain. Also, do you remember when we talked about how someone with autism learns better by doing? This means that if you try to teach your child to tie his shoes and just show him how to do it, he will have difficulty mirroring the movements. Instead, guide him step by step, placing each of his fingers in the right place. This will take advantage of his muscle memory, making the learning process much more concrete.

Thermoception — temperature perception

Heat hypersensitivity, also known as heat intolerance, means you tend to feel uncomfortable in hot weather.

When you have autism, "uncomfortable" doesn't even begin to describe how heat makes you feel. Summer can become a season of misery.

When you are feeling cold, you can always wear an extra layer of clothes but dealing with heat is more problematic. So, don't be surprised if your child becomes lethargic on hotter days, moving as little as possible — after all, movement generates heat. An air conditioner is helpful, but the additional noise can be troublesome if the child also has sound hypersensitive.

Cold hypersensitivity, more commonly known as cold intolerance, as the name implies, refers to the opposite problem. Someone intolerant to cold may end up walking around dressed up as if he was living in the Arctic Circle, especially if he lives in a cold or damp area.

At the same time, in cases of cold hyposensitivity, the person with autism can be seen wearing a loose t-shirt while everyone else is holding tight to their coat and scarf.

When it comes to temperature perception, parents need to be especially alert in the cases of heat intolerance, making sure their children remain cool.

A note on neuroplasticity and desensitization therapy

Our brain is plastic. It adapts. Just because someone is oversensitive to a certain sound frequency now, it doesn't mean he will stay that way forever.

For example, many factors influence a person's degree of sensory sensitivity, including how they feel and their level of physical and mental fatigue. This means that a sound volume that was okay yesterday might be painful today.

Besides that, other factors such as the degree of control someone has over the source of the sound, also affect your sensory tolerance.

As an example, suppose I'm oversensitive to low bass frequencies. If you come into the room and turn on the stereo, you might hear me telling you to turn down the volume. However, if I'm the one in control, maybe I'd tolerate the sound for a few extra seconds.

Now here's the key idea: controlled exposition builds up your tolerance. Something similar happens with phobias. If I'm afraid of snakes and you force me to touch one, I'll panic and my phobia will get much worse. However, if I'm the one controlling my level of proximity to the snake things will be different.

Imagine I decide to stay within ten feet of the snake. I'm sweating, I'm afraid, I want to run away. But through sheer willpower, I choose to stay there. Over time, my heart rate decreases, my thoughts calm down. What's happening? Before, my brain believed:

- "Snake means danger. Stay as far as you can from a snake. Always."

However, after getting used to remaining within 10 feet of a snake my brain adapted, it evolved, it now believes:

- "Snake means danger. But, if I remain at least 10 feet away, I'm safe."

Given enough time and opportunities for this kind of controlled exposition, I may even end up deciding to touch the snake.

The take home point is this: persuade your child to test his limits. Make it a game. "Let's try to break the world record!" See if he can challenge himself to listen to a certain sound for a few more seconds.

Since your child knows that as soon as the volume hurts his ears or becomes uncomfortable, he can lower it or turn it off immediately, he's more willing to give it a try and his tolerance will also tend to be greater.

Change won't happen overnight, but given sufficient time, hypersensitivities may get better. A gradual exposure, always under the control of the person with hypersensitivity, can have beneficial effects on the brain's ability to tolerate stimuli. It's a desensitization therapy.

The opposite is also true.

For example, people with photosensitivity usually wear sunglasses. This causes their hypersensitivity to increase. Likewise, if someone with sound hypersensitivity often wears earplugs, over time, his sensitivity to sound increases.

In any case, dealing with unpleasant sensory stimuli for a long time will lead to sensory overload. What is it?

Sensory Overload

When someone with autism has to deal with sensory stimuli to which they are hypersensitive, this leads to discomfort and stimming.

If this is happening because you are forcing the person to remain there, this will have a negative impact on your relationship.

Do this often and the autistic person will feel disgusted at you. Don't take this likely. If you blast your car radio with a person with sound hypersensitivity next to you, you'll be torturing him. Do this enough times and just the thought of being with you again will cause the autistic person to stim in despair.

At the same time, demanding an autistic person to stay in a movie theater, shopping mall, or other places, when the person has already exceeded his ability to deal with sensory stimuli, will overwhelm him. This is called sensory overload, and it's a serious problem.

To gain a deeper understanding of the phenomenon of sensory overload, consider the following, imagine that you've spent several days living in a pitch-dark basement. Then, you decide to leave on a bright, sunny day. Once the light hits your eyes, how do you feel? This is what the autistic person feels when he's overwhelmed by sensory stimuli.

How does an autistic person deal with sensory overload? By using the tool he knows best: stimming. But what if stimming isn't enough to calm him down? If no one removes him to a place free from sensory stimulation, the autistic person will have a nervous breakdown. These crises are very specific and are called meltdowns. In the next chapter, we will look at what a meltdown is and what can be done to alleviate it when it arises.

Chapter 7

How to Identify and Stop a Meltdown?

For the past few weeks, your son with Asperger's syndrome hasn't stopped talking about the new superhero movie. Now, you and your family are finally sitting in the theater and he is elated.

Unfortunately, the movie falls short of his expectations. He's sad and disappointed. These sensations dance within him as he shakes his legs, attempting to tame the emotional discomfort.

On the way back, you turn the radio on and try to cheer up your two children. But the volume is a bit too high. You attempt to engage your son with Asperger's, but he is irritated and responds badly.

Upon arriving home, things don't get any better. "Josh, I need you to clean your room," you tell him. "But mother, I don't feel like it!" He replies in a tone of disgust. "Josh, we agreed we would go to the movie that you both wanted to see and that when we arrived you would clean your room. You promised me this, Josh, now you have to comply," you reply, irritated.

Out of nowhere, Josh explodes, runs to the bedroom, slamming the door behind him.

What just happened?

A meltdown. As we've learned in the introduction of the book, this term, meltdown, is used to describe two things:

- the intensity of an autistic breakdown

- the fission of a nuclear reactor.

Do you remember the connection between these two points?

As a parent or educator, watching a child beating himself, screaming or even throwing things, can be as scary and confusing as witnessing the fission of a nuclear reactor.

How can you deal with something like that? To overcome this obstacle, we'll divide it into five questions and we'll analyze each one of them. The five questions are:

- What is a meltdown?

- What causes the meltdown?

- How can you know if a meltdown is about to happen?

- How do you prevent a meltdown from occurring?

- How can you deal with a meltdown once it begins?

What is a meltdown?

Our brain is designed to analyze the environment around us for signs of danger. Whenever the brain detects a threat, our body is transformed. We become more alert, fast and strong.

Why?

Because the extra adrenaline, along with the other stress hormones, causes several changes within us.

We call this process the stress response. This is an emergency mode. We turn into a kind of superhuman. Surely, you've been through this.

For example, when we are afraid or angry, our heart beats faster, our breathing rate increases, and our muscles tighten. Our body isn't just preparing to fight, it's preparing to win the battle.

Among all these changes, there're some affecting how we process information. When we are in danger our mind focuses on the threat we're facing until it's resolved. In normal situations, this is very useful. After all, if we are being chased by a fierce animal it makes sense for our brain to focus on the problem until we're safe again.

However, the stress response can become problematic. This happens when it is activated to help us deal with problems that can't be solved by force alone.

For example, if the autistic person is dealing with a loud noise, something that causes pain in his ears, his body will activate the stress response. His heart will beat harder and his body will transform to overcome the situation. His mind will focus on the loud noise and the solution: getting out of there.

But there's a problem. Due to communication difficulties between the various neural networks, the stress response can get out of control.

To illustrate, imagine two situations involving someone with a neurotypical brain. Notice how both situations cause the activation of the stress response but in different degrees:

Situation 1:

You are in the supermarket line and the young cashier is taking some time due to his inexperience. You are in a hurry. You try to be understanding, but you are watching the minutes fly by. This is a problem. Your brain detects this threat and pumps adrenaline into your blood. This causes your body to prepare for battle. From 1 to 10 your stress response is at level 3.

Unpleasant, it's true, but you can still control yourself. This isn't a situation that can be resolved by force, so you keep your cool.

Then, a man asks you permission to pass, but when you give him just enough room, so he can advance to the other side of the supermarket, he pretends he'll move forward but stops, right in front of you! You've just been deceived.

Now your body is boiling with stress.

Images of war move through your head and you can barely dominate them. From 1 to 10, we would say that this situation is an 8. Fortunately, you exercise self-control and avoid open war.

Situation 2:

You're leaving the bank with your monthly income, making the mistake of counting the money in the middle of the street. Soon enough, two hooded men are threatening you with knives. Immediately, your heart explodes, flooding your muscles with adrenaline-rich blood. One moment later, your unconscious mind gives you back control over your thoughts. Now, it's up to you to decide what to do next.

Do you fight, surrender your money or run away?

If you decide to either fight or flee, your body is fully prepared to give your muscles the energy and the oxygen they need to respond to your request.

Luckily you can control yourself just enough to resist the urge to react. After all, your physical integrity is worth far more than any sum of money. You give them the money and the thieves walk away. Gradually you calm yourself down.

However, from 1 to 10, while those knives were pointed at you, you had your stress response at 10.

Once the robbers are out of sight, it lowers to a 6.

Did you notice what happened?

In each case, your body prepared you for war. This happened automatically and at an unconscious level.

This stress response is controlled by our limbic system. It's a process over which we have no control. It's our brain the one deciding, in a moment's notice, whether the stress response will be activated and at what level this activation will occur.

However, did you notice what happened right after it was activated?

The final decision on what to do was given to the conscious mind. This area, responsible for decision making, is called the prefrontal cortex.

It's through this area that we exercise self-control and regulate our impulses, even when under extreme pressure to fight or flee.

However, how would things have been if the communication between the limbic system and the prefrontal cortex was damaged? This is what happens in autism. With what result?

Again, the answer is "it depends," since every person with autism is affected differently. But, in general, this is what happens when someone has autism:

- The stress response tends to be activated much more often and intensely.

- Communication between the limbic system and the prefrontal cortex does not occur as clearly, preventing the person from fully understanding what's happening to his body, and making it difficult to exercise self-control.

In the case of someone with autism, even a simple situation may end up triggering a level 9 or 10 stress response. With what result?

Since the person with autism has trouble controlling himself through internal means, he tries to calm his limbic system externally through stimming. But stimming is limited in its ability to reduce the intensity of the stress response. With what result?

A nervous breakdown, or meltdown. This nervous breakdown can include panic, a rage, vomiting, crying, and despair, or even push the person into a state of inanimation as if his brain had shut down.

It all depends on the emotions behind the stress response.

For example, in the case of the line-cutter, the unfairness of the situation could cause a rage meltdown. The injustice of the situation would lead our limbic system to prepare the body to fight for the reestablishment of justice. This anger could easily rise to level 10, along with the support of an equally strong, level 10, stress response.

Now, imagine if the line-cutter looked back at the autistic person with a wicked grin. The autistic person could simply not be able to control the urge to react, either through his words or more violently.

Likewise, intense fear coupled with an intense stress response would trigger a panic attack faster in the autistic than in the neurotypical person. Once again, due to the autistic's difficulties in exercising self-control.

Moreover, sudden sadness could lead to a bout of depression. This state of depression could take several days to pass or end up turning into clinical depression.

Extreme disgust, on the other hand, could lead to nausea and vomiting. In the same way, if something surprises the autistic person to a very high degree he may become paralyzed and shut down, not for a few minutes, but for several hours.

At the same time, if several intense emotions occur together, followed by the activation of the stress response, this would trigger a kind of meltdown combining the characteristics of these various types of nervous breakdowns we've been describing.

All these because of the miscommunication between the limbic system, the prefrontal cortex and all the other areas of the brain involved in emotional intelligence.

What causes the meltdown?

In someone with autism, a meltdown is triggered by the accumulation of stressful situations. These include:

- Anything that activates the unique sensory hypersensitivities of the person.

- Dealing with people.

- Unexpected changes in routine.

- Having too much new information to process.

- All the other common situations that even a neurotypical would find stressful.

Stimming can delay a meltdown but isn't a sure way to prevent it.

Imagine a scale from 0 to 100. This scale represents how close we are to a meltdown. The autistic person starts his day at 0. Eventually, stresses build up. The irritating noise of a passing motorcycle (+ 5 points per each second of noise), the flickering lights in the room (+10 points for every 15 minutes in the room), having to interact with one person for 20 minutes (+10 points). An unexpected change of plans (+20 points). Finding out that, after all, he won't have the opportunity to be alone to relax and recharge his mental energy (+30 points). Did you notice how easily we're getting to 100?

By then, people around the person are already commenting on the weird way he's rocking in his chair — which, by the way, is reducing his stress level by 10 points per minute.

In fact, the autistic is doing everything he can to avoid a meltdown. However, if stressful situations continue to accumulate, the number of stress points will eventually rise above 100 and a meltdown will occur.

The good news is that, after the meltdown, we are back at 0.

However, the person will feel ashamed and their self-esteem will be very low. Also, going through a meltdown is a disturbing experience.

As a man with autism expressed himself:

> « In the case of extreme sensory overload, I have to deal with suicidal thoughts. It really is that awful. »

How can you know if a meltdown is about to happen?

Stimming is an effective way to monitor your child's stress level. Even though he may seem calm and relaxed, if he's shaking his leg or pounding his fingers on the table, he isn't. Inside there's emotional agitation. Stimming is helping him keeping this turmoil in check. It's also warning you things aren't as calm as they seem.

Never ignore the message behind stimming.

Even a serene facial expression is unreliable. In autism, the areas responsible for facial expressions don't work in the same way as in a neurotypical person. This means that the emotions the person is feeling don't always show up. In fact, the opposite occurs. Someone with autism can end up laughing with sadness, causing embarrassment, for example, at a funeral.

If your child is stimming, you have to put on your detective hat. Something is causing the stimming behavior.

- Is it some noise that your neurotypical brain has already learned to ignore, but which your child's brain has no ability to disregard?

- Is it some concern?

- Is it a sign that he has already reached his limit of interaction with other people?

- Does he need help to deal with any routine changes?
- Is it too hot or too cold?

- Is he feeling any pain or other physical distress?

- Is he bored?

If you can pinpoint the root cause, you'll be better equipped to prevent a future meltdown.

How do you prevent a meltdown from occurring?

There are several ways to prevent a meltdown:

1. **Eliminate what you think might be causing sensory distress.** Help your child take off any clothes that may be making him itch or warming him too much. Turn off any flickering lights. Turn off the music and reduce other noises as much as possible. Remove objects with bright colors or patterns from his vicinity.

2. **Take your child to a place without people.** A room that he knows and where he has control over his environment, ideally his bedroom.

3. **Let him distract himself with some hobby or activity that he loves.**

4. **Help him find a place where he can do all the stimming he wants.**

5. **Talk to him in a soothing voice.** This is comforting even if your child doesn't understand everything you are saying.

6. **Apply pressure on his body by hugging him tightly.** Remember, however, that he must have full control over how much pressure you are exerting on him and for how long. Otherwise, the pressure may have the opposite effect. Therefore, if you hug your child, be aware of any sign of him pushing you.

Likewise, there are things that, if done when he's on the verge of a meltdown, will only make things worse, hastening the meltdown and its intensity. These things include:

1. **Punish your child.** This will only activate the stress response even more.

2. **Make him interact with people.** This is one of the most effective ways to mentally exhaust an autistic person.

3. **Ask questions that require him to think things through to answer.** This type of questions requires a kind of mental focus that causes physiological changes similar to the stress response. Just imagine how you'd feel if you're asked to solve a challenging math problem when you're tired.

4. **Force him to adapt to a change in routine.** Remember that he will only adapt when he has had enough time to imagine himself going through the new situation. This

implies that he should be given access to the maximum amount of information about what will happen.

5. Ignore sensory hypersensitivities and sensory overload.

Over time you will gain a good sense of what disturbs your child and you will be able to distinguish between the regular stimming he does to soothe himself and the emergency stimming that occurs before a meltdown. Also, as you keep on learning about the inner workings of your child's stimming behavior, you will be better equipped to distinguish a meltdown from a tantrum.

A meltdown always has a logical cause related to an inability to exercise control over the limbic system. A tantrum is a strategy the child uses to get his way.

How can you deal with a meltdown once it begins?

Do your best to move your child to the most neutral environment possible. The best place in the world is his room. Why? Because he has control over his environment. He can stim at will and he's near his favorite things. Unfortunately, many meltdowns occur outside your home. Or, even if they happen indoors, they occur due to factors inside the person's body. Disturbing emotions cause a kind of turbulence coming from within and outside of your direct control.

However, don't despair. Just the fact that you are worried and trying to do what you can has a positive effect on your child, conveying him a sense of peace and security. Over time, this will create a stronger connection between you. A unique bond. It is very unlikely that he will ever find someone else attempting to meet his special needs with such affection and goodwill.

Even if he can't express it, he feels your love and you can be sure this love is reciprocated.

That's when something magical happens.

In the literature on autism, there are many references to the so-called "favorite people." A favorite person is any person who gives mental energy to the autistic rather than withdrawing it from him. Does that sound unscientific and dubious to you?

My experience says otherwise.

In fact, this subject is so vital that it deserves its own chapter.

In any case, look at a meltdown as yet another opportunity to strengthen the special bond between you and someone with autism. Be that unique person who actually gets him.

Chapter 8

Favorite People — Myth or Reality?

We all have people we like better than others. Most never become more than acquaintances. Some become friends, but very few become blood brothers. However, when this happens, our life improves.

Imagine the situations we've described earlier. You're in the supermarket line, disturbed by the line-cutter in front of you. Then, you see your best friend enter through the supermarket door. He's someone who understands you and is always supportive. He is a kind, friendly, intelligent and mature person. Positive adjectives can't describe how much you appreciate this person. When you see him you feel better, it's like if your limbic system said to itself:

"Well, now that my friend is here, I no longer have to fight alone. This means I can't reduce the level of my stress response."

This kind of close connection is often observed in happy couples. They love each other, and a healthy interdependence has developed between them.

When he is around she feels relaxed and confident. It seems that difficulties don't affect her as much. When she's around, he's even more motivated to deal with problems and face any challenges.

The same happens between neurotypical children and their loving parents. For example, when a son sees his father entering through the school gate he knows that the bullies no longer have any power over him.

Furthermore, this healthy interdependence is also observed in completely different areas of life. For example, a firefighter develops a strong sense of brotherhood towards his companions. These men know that their lives are in each other's hands. Over the years, they have lived the "no man is left behind" motto so much that they have created a strong bond. Sometimes, this connection is stronger than family ties.

What do all these bonds have in common?

All these bonds have in common people caring for one another. This is a cycle. If I pay attention to your needs with the goal of fulfilling them, you have the tendency to do the same for me. It's a win-win situation.

In the case of autism, their needs are very special. That's why we need to be even more alert. But the effort pays off.

When you systematically pay attention and care for the special needs of someone with autism, their limbic system — the same responsible for the unconscious detection of threats — learns that you are synonymous with understanding, comfort, and protection.

That makes perfect sense. After all, suppose I have autism and loud noises drive me insane. In this case, if my mother always covers my ears with her hands until I calm myself down, it doesn't take me long to learn that "mother" equals "relief."

Moreover, if when I'm afraid my mother talks to me in a soothing tone, helping me to process the information, how long do you think it'll take for my limbic system to associate "mother" with comfort and protection?

People with autism aren't stupid. Yes, several areas inside their brain don't operate in a typical way, and the communication lines between them may not be working well, but they do know how to distinguish between someone who relieves their pain and someone who doesn't.

Over time, these caring people become the so-called "favorite people". This means that the autistic person is much more tolerant of their proximity, often wishing that they be present, for their simple presence is soothing to them and gives them strength instead of wearing them down.

How do you become a favorite person?

Maybe so far you have tried to love your autistic child in the same way you love your neurotypical children. This may work to some extent, but if you then ignore the effect shopping centers and other noisy places have on your child, or if you force him to endure clothes that scratch his skin, all your efforts may fall to the ground.

Not that your child wants to ignore all the good you do for him. It's just that, from the perspective of his brain, you are an unreliable source of comfort.

For example, imagine that during the car ride the volume of the radio starts affecting your child. When he complains about it, and everyone starts saying it should be even higher, what do you do? If you ignore his protests and turn the volume up, he will learn that sometimes nobody cares about his needs, not even his parent. Even though he may never verbalize it, that's how he feels.

On the other hand, if you always care about his needs, the end result will be much different. When he's in a different car, and people react badly to his requests to lower the volume, he'll think, "I wish my mother were here" instead of thinking, "I wish I were alone."

In the case of children with Asperger, being a favorite person means that you will become the target of their long discourses on his favorite topics. But this is a small price to pay in exchange for the strong bond that will develop. And look on the bright side: in time you will become an expert on his favorite topics.

Changes in routine and the favorite person

Throughout the book, we have talked about the negative impact a routine change can have on a person with autism. We have seen how this is true even with more moderate forms of autism, such as Asperger's syndrome. Why does this happen?

Due to its configuration, the autistic brain needs more time to process some types of information, such as abstract data or information with social-emotional content.

Accordingly, when a routine change involves these types of information, the person needs an unusual amount of time to analyze it.

For example, imagine that a young man with autism is asked to go and get some groceries from the store. At first, he doesn't want to go. He even feels some disgust at the idea of going. Then he stims while trying to force himself to go. He keeps imagining himself performing the task, trying to predict all that can go wrong and how he could handle it. He prepares himself mentally to deal with the sensory sensitivities he expects to find in the grocery store. After a few minutes, or hours, he is ready.

This process required a considerable amount of mental effort and was somewhat exhausting. But now it's over. He is ready and, if you were to ask him, he might tell you he's feeling a certain newfound enthusiasm with the idea of going.

In the meantime, this young man's father is thinking, "Well, I know how my son hates crowded places. I will let him know I'll be the one going to the grocery store. I think I'm just going to ask him to clean his bedroom."

Dad hopes this will make his son happy. After all, this reassignment of chores seems to account for his son's special needs. What could go wrong?

But, as soon as the boy realizes how his routine has been changed, again, he closes himself in his bedroom, angry and in meltdown, stimming away his distress. The father is left in shock, unable to understand what happened. "Why is my son so hard to please?" he asks himself, saddened.

What went wrong?

After readying himself for a task, a routine change may spend even more mental energy than actually going and performing the task.

Why?

Because now, his mental energy will seem to have been used up in vain. Also, he will have to deal with the disappointment of no longer going to the supermarket. In addition, he'll now have to force himself to process each step required by the new task.

For all these reasons, it's important to talk things through with the autistic person, trying to understand how he feels about the change in routine.

Whenever possible, let him know well in advance of any changes in his daily routine. Maybe you're thinking, "But if I let him know in advance, he'll just spend more time stressing about it."

Maybe. But he'll also have extra time to rehearse everything in his mind.

You have two options. You can make him feel the pain of a routine change all at once, potentially provoking a meltdown, or you can spread this pain throughout many hours, or days, making it feel more like an annoying but manageable ache.

Besides, by applying the suggestions found in Chapter 4 you can do a lot to minimize his emotional distress.

Will you become a favorite person?

Yew, you will. After all, you took the time to read this entire book. This alone is evidence of your loving interest in people with autism. They are very lucky to have you in their life. It is this love that will motivate you to put into practice the suggestions in this book, even when it's difficult to do so.

What if you make mistakes?

This is normal and expected. But before we consider how to deal with mistakes, it's interesting that John Gottman, a psychology professor and author of several books on relationships, speaks about the 5:1 rule for couples.

This rule states that to compensate for a bad action, you must do 5 good actions.

This happens because of the way our limbic system is built. The areas of our brain responsible for detecting threats give much more weight to a bad action than to a good one.

For example, suppose a dog is friendly for a while but then bites me. Do I go home thinking, "What a nice dog, it was so sweet for most of the time"? No.

The same is true of traumas.

Maybe I spent my life taking the elevator without any problem. But, getting stuck in a broken elevator for a few hours and my opinion on their safety changes considerably.

Using an elevator remains as safe after I got stuck as it was before. In fact, what is the likelihood of someone getting stuck twice? We can say that it is smaller than getting stuck once in a lifetime. But our limbic system thinks otherwise.

Before elevators were safe, now they aren't. End of story.

Something similar happens when dealing with others.

If someone treats us bad a few times in a row, we begin to gain some aversion for that person. To turn this negative opinion into a more balanced viewpoint requires an effort to express empathy. We must keep asking ourselves:

- Why did he act like this?

- Was he tired or worried?

- If I were in the same situation, what guarantees me that I wouldn't end up doing the same or worse?

- Haven't I done similar things before? Does this prove that I am a bad person? Then, why should his incorrect action be enough to prove that he is a bad person?

- What are his qualities?

- Does he lack qualities, or do I just not know him well enough?

- If I don't know him, who am I mad at?

Our brain is designed to pay more attention to bad things than to good things. This means we need to make a conscious effort and resist our tendency to judge them as evil.

As per John Gottman's rule, this person will need to make us 5 times more good actions just so our brain stops seeing him as a potential threat.

And when we are the person who treated the other badly?

Helping the person process what happened it's essential.

For example, imagine that the dog that bit me could speak. Suppose he would come to my house and explain that he bit me because I had injured him upon squeezing his neck. He then proceeds to explain to me his temperament problems and apologizes.

Over the next few days, I notice how this dog makes every effort to treat me right. Over time my opinion starts to change.

Maybe I'll start thinking, "Well, maybe that was a one-time occurrence. The truth is, I really squeezed him that day. Besides, he didn't even actually bite me, he just laid his teeth on my hand. The truth is, I scratched my hand on his teeth when I pulled it out."

Similarly, if we did something that hurt an autistic person, it's important to apologize and try to explain what happened — in a way adapted to the person's degree of autism.

In any case, over time, good actions will speak louder than any wrong we have done before.

After all, if you are a parent, you still have the task of educating your child with autism. This involves giving proper discipline whenever appropriate. In addition, a good parent has good reasons not to do or give the child everything he wants.

Just make sure that when disciplining your child, you consider his special needs. For example, if you tell someone with autism that he is a bad person he will interpret this literally. After all, his thinking his concrete.

The expression "you are a bad person" will fill his mind with images of what it means to be bad. Hence, he will associate all these images with himself. He loves you, so your opinion will have an impact on him.

What can you do?

Be specific. Discipline the child by telling him what specific action was bad. Explain to him how the action made you feel and describe how he should have behaved.

Because of the way his brain is set up to think concretely, telling the autistic exactly what was expected of him, step by step — if possible in writing — is far more effective than telling him what he shouldn't have done.

How to communicate with someone with autism?

To illustrate, suppose you want your child to clean the room. Notice what would not work:

"This room is a mess."

For the autistic mind, this statement is regarded and registered as an opinion. "My father thinks my room is a mess."

"I want this room shinning!" wouldn't work either.

What does "shinning" even mean? This word is abstract. Maybe, from your concrete thinking child point of view, it's already shinning.

In addition, thinking about each of the many steps involved in the task may end up making the autistic person view the task of arranging the room as extraordinarily difficult. The equivalent of you getting close to your neurotypical son and telling him, "Go change the oil in the car." Your neurotypical son would feel surprised at the request, not knowing where to start, or what to do.

Moreover, the angry tone in your voice could trigger anxiety, even panic.

So, what to do?

Be as concrete and direct as possible. Show what you want to be done, step by step.

"First, I need you to get up, pick up the clothes on the floor and pile them up right here where I'm standing. Then, you have to move the clothes to the laundry basket. Next, pick up your toys from the floor and put them on the shelves in any way you want. Do the same for any other items or objects. In the end, pick up the broom and sweep the room. "

Ideally, exemplify to him what each task involves. Also, since he learns best by doing, guide him through each step.

And don't forget the written list. It may seem crazy to give a child a list of the steps needed to do something as simple as cleaning the room. But all these are measures that facilitate his work.

Tip: Google the task. You' usually find at least a step-by-step list you can print out. Sites like www.wikihow.com provide such lists, often with colorful pictures.

Then, if he refuses to perform the task you can decide to discipline him in any way you deem appropriate. For example: "Until you follow these steps thoroughly, you won't be allowed to play any video games." This is a reasonable request with an equally balanced consequence.

Again, each case is a case. No two autistics are alike. It all depends on the degree of autism and the special needs, sensibilities and unique personality that your child has. A personality that exists along with autism and is as unique as that of any other person.

Over time you'll find that certain tasks cause too much discomfort to your child. As the loving parent you are — or else you would not be bothering to read this — surely you will know how to adapt your requests to your child's unique difficulties.

To illustrate, if dealing with detergent causes olfactory sensitivities to your child, you may choose to buy neutral detergents or let your child choose which odors he tolerates best. Otherwise, you may decide that any tasks requiring the use of cleaning agents will always be done by you or your wife. Maybe you'll also choose to do them while your child is away from home, and there's enough time for the smells to dissipate before he returns.

In the next chapter, we will take a closer look at the various special needs we've considered throughout this book. We'll also be looking at specific strategies you can implement to meet these special needs.

Chapter 9

Special Needs of the Autistic and How to Meet Them

No one really understands what causes autism. Due to genetic and environmental factors, the brain doesn't develop in a typical way. Some researchers propose that deficiencies in some key nutrients during pregnancy and the child's early years, such as vitamin D, are associated with the development of a brain with autism.

Others suggest that the problem is in the digestive tract. Inadequate metabolism of key nutrients during the brain's development prevent it from receiving adequate nourishment for it to develop correctly. Even others suggest a possible relationship between exposure to heavy metals and autism.

Some argue that there is a link between vaccines and autism. This is a topic where there're very strong opinions on both sides of the issue. This is understandable, and a detailed analysis of this subject is beyond the scope of this book. If the reader has information on this topic, which make you choose either side of the debate, I'd like to examine it. You can contact me at tiagohenriques@academiaciencia.com

One thing, however, is certain: there is no consensus on the causes of autism. It's possible that autism has multiple causes. After all, anything that influences brain development can cause autism and there are countless factors with the potential to affect the brain and its growth.

However, most agree that because of his atypical brain, someone with autism processes reality in a different way. That is where this book and my experience aim to help you.

What happens is that the neural networks are all there, but they don't work in an ordinary way.

What is claimed by some researchers, such as Temple Grandin, is that someone on the spectrum has a higher amount of cables within the areas, or neural modules, but a lower amount of nerve fibers linking them together. In addition, this person has comparatively few nerve fibers, or "electric cables," connecting the various areas to the prefrontal cortex — the decision-making area.

This means that the conscious mind receives incomplete information about what is going on in the rest of the brain while, at the same time, having a limited ability to influence what is happening in these same areas.

The diagnosis

It depends a lot on the expertise of the professional doing the analysis. But, as a general rule, the diagnosis of autism occurs when someone has difficulties in the following aspects:

1. Sensorial processing.

2. Emotional processing.

3. Social processing and theory of mind.

4. Communication.

5. Executive functions.

Depending on his degree of difficulties in one, or more, of these aspects, the person may even end up receiving an incorrect diagnosis, as we will see later.

For now, the important point to keep in mind is that each of these aspects is dependent on a specific area, or areas, within the brain.

Now, as we recapitulate each of these aspects, we will try to do so in a concrete way.

To do this, we will imagine that the areas of the brain responsible for processing each of these aspects are trying to answer some questions they constantly ask themselves.

In this way, we can consider that having problems in one of these five aspects involves having difficulties in (1) **getting answers to the questions** that the areas of the brain are asking themselves, (2) **transmitting these answers** to the other areas and (3) **adjusting behavioral responses according to the answers they've found.**

This means we can define "degree of autism" as "the degree to which these three difficulties affect someone's life." Confused by all the abstract talk? Don't worry. We will now be making a concrete analysis of this subject.

1. Sensory Processing

This type of processing occurs as our brain tries to get answers to the following questions:

- What information is entering the brain through each of the internal sensors and each of the sensory organs?

- What am I seeing, hearing, smelling, touching and tasting?

- What is the temperature of my body?

- What is my degree of pain?

- What are the location, inclination, and acceleration of the limbs?

- What's the degree of contraction and relaxation of each muscle group?

- How intense are these sensations?

- How should they be interpreted?

2. Emotional processing

This type of processing involves answering the following questions:

- What are my needs?

- Do I have the means (resources) to satisfy them?

- How should I adapt to ensure that I can meet them?

- What are the sensations present in my body?

- What do they mean?

- How should I react to them?

3. Social processing and theory of mind

The term "theory of mind" refers to the human ability to understand that other people are different from us. Their mind is unique. These are the questions our brain is trying to answer as it processes social information:

- Who is this other human being that I have detected in my environment?

- What is he feeling?

- What is he communicating through his words?

- What is he thinking and not communicating openly?

- What are his intentions?

- What are his needs?

- Is he a threat to me?

- How should I react to him?

Someone with autism has many difficulties in this domain of theory of mind. For example, when I'm alone I eat with my mouth open and I'm fine with that. After all, I don't see the food being chewed through my open mouth. However, if you are across the table you can see the chewed food through my open mouth.

Having the capacity of theory of mind fully functional means that I can make the connection: If I feel disgusted when I see other people eating with their mouths open, it stands to reason that other people will also feel the same way about my habit of eating with my mouth open.

In contrast, someone with a limited theory of mind might come to a completely different conclusion. "I don't feel disgusted when I eat with my mouth open, therefore, you won't either."

This brain failed to make a seemingly simple connection: "If it makes me feel this way, it's likely that if I do the same to others, it will also affect them in a similar way."

As someone with Asperger's Syndrome expressed himself:

« I don't like being interrupted, but I interrupt others all the time. I've never really thought about it, but the truth is that if I don't like being interrupted, it's only natural that others don't like it when I interrupt them. I used to think: "People's reaction when I interrupt them amuses me, so it's only natural that they find it funny too. »

If someone lacking theory of mind isn't helped to gain a more balanced perspective, he will assume that the reaction he's having at that moment is the same reaction that other people are having.

This means that when he eats with his mouth open, he thinks, "This doesn't affect me, so it surely isn't affecting others." However, when you are the one eating with your mouth open, he reasons: "This disgusts me. Surely it's disgusting everyone else too."

Because of this, theory of mind is closely linked with empathy.

4. Communication

This aspect is closely related to social processing. Here, several areas of the brain come together to try to extract information from the sensory stimuli picked up by the eyes and ears:

- Are these sounds noise or do they contain information?

- To what kind of concepts is the information referring to?

- How does it relate to what I already know?

- How should this new information influence what I already know?

- What's the tone of voice?

- How does it modify what is being communicated?

- What are his facial expressions?

- What's his body language?

- Is this person being ironic or sarcastic?

- Is there humor in what was said?

- Is he telling the truth or lying?

- Is he silent because he's finished communicating or because he's thinking about what he'll say next?

5. Executive functions

We rarely hear the term "executive functions." However, they are indispensable. They include the ability to block an urge to do something, plan things, control our thoughts, modulate our emotions and ignore intrusive sensory stimuli.

All these functions require good communication between the whole brain:

- Should I continue to pay attention to this sensory stimulus?

- Is what I'm feeling appropriate?

- Is the degree of these emotions adequate?

- Does it make sense to worry about this?

- Should I prevent this emotion from intensifying?

- How can I solve this problem?

- What is the end result I intend to achieve?

- What is the next step?

- What resources can I use?

- If I don't have one of the resources, how can I get it?

Defining "Autism" in concrete terms

Taking each of these 5 aspects into consideration, the greater the difficulty a brain has to (1) get answers to the questions each brain area asks, (2) transmit these answers to the other areas and (3) adjust his behavior accordingly, the greater the degree of autism.

Of course, none of us is perfect. Hardly anyone can exercise full control over their emotions. But in some cases, this difficulty causes multiple problems.

Usually, when defining the degree of autism, much attention is given to aspects number 3, 4 and 5 (Social Processing and Theory of Mind, Communication, and Executive functions). After all, if someone has their neural networks damaged to a point where they can't communicate or can't inhibit impulses, this causes many more difficulties than if one has only difficulty expressing empathy.

Thus, the diagnosis of the depth of autism is mainly related to the difficulties in these aspects.

Aspects number 1 and 2 (Sensory Processing and Emotional Processing) are sometimes ignored, even though they cause a lot of suffering to the person. As we have seen, sensory overload can even lead to suicidal thoughts. In addition, the greater the difficulty in controlling unpleasant emotions, such as fear, anger, and disgust, the lower the quality of life.

In the same way, when difficulties in inhibiting anger (Aspect 5) and a lack in theory of mind (Aspect 3) come together, they will cause intense interpersonal problems.

Because of all these incongruencies in diagnosis, someone with a deeper form of autism can benefit a lot from the help of knowledgeable relatives, educators, and others with more moderate forms of autism. These helping hand will make all the difference in the quality of life of someone with profound autism.

What are the special needs of someone with autism?

We can divide the special needs of someone with autism into 5 (not directly related to the 5 aspects mentioned above). They are:

A. Processing Information

B. Controlling Emotions

C. Protecting Oneself from Sensory Hypersensitivity

D. Resting

E. Feeling Support

These are human needs, common to each one of us. So, why do we say that in the case of someone with autism they are special?

Because the strategies used to meet these needs are uncommon. In fact, as we have seen, sometimes, the same strategies that would help a neurotypical person backfire when tried on someone with autism.

To illustrate the point, let us consider our common need to eat. Not everyone can eat the same things. Someone who's allergic to peanuts can't use "eating peanut butter" as a strategy to satisfy his need to feed himself. If he does so, he will suffer the consequences. Does that make him subhuman? Does it tell us anything about the real character of this person? No.

Similarly, someone with a faster metabolism needs to regularly eat, while someone else with may decide to modify his eating habits due to a disease or to lose weight.

There is the same basic need in all these cases: eating. But, for the most diverse circumstances, this need must be met with different strategies, performed at varying times and intensities.

Likewise, visiting a place full of people can be an excellent strategy to distract and calm down a neurotypical child, but it could end up triggering a meltdown in someone with autism.

With this in mind, what are the appropriate strategies to meet the special needs that someone with autism has?

A. Understanding the Need to Process Information from the Point of View of Someone with Autism

This is a complex topic, so we'll begin with an illustration. In the end, you'll have learned all about this first special need.

Consider the subject of dating.

When a neurotypical boy is in love with a girl he'll spend many hours thinking about each word the girl says to him. He'll probably go online and type: "What does it mean when a girl blush while talking to you?" and "Signs of romantic interest."

From each new interaction with the girl, the boy will extract new bits of information to analyze.

We can imagine each new bit of information as a single puzzle piece. When new pieces don't fit in the puzzle, he feels anxious. Does he need to tear the puzzle apart and start all over again?

For example, for the past two weeks, the girl has been making eye contact with him each time they see each other in the school hallway. Once, he even mustered the courage to smile at her, and she smiled back!

Each of these pieces is coming together to construct an image of a reality where she's in love with him.

But when he tried to engage her in a dialogue yesterday, she ignored him. What a disappointment. Now he's back to the drawing board. Does she love him or not? It seems he'll never know for sure.

In contrast, months from now, when he asks her out and she finally says "yes" with a big smile, he'll feel confident and at peace. The puzzle will be completed... for a few days. The real world never stops sending him new bits of information, so the puzzle never really ends.

However, even though there's always this looming possibility that our conclusions are incorrect, mental clarity is of the utmost importance for the human brain. Fortunately, this sense of clarity comes, not when the puzzle is completed, but when we've built it just enough to have a clear, logical, and concrete picture of the subject we are considering.

Dating is a great example. Why?

Because both a neurotypical and an autistic boy will have trouble understanding if the girl loves them or not. Both will spend many hours revisiting memories, obsessing over the subject, trying to complete their puzzle. Both will daydream about it. That's how infatuation works in humans.

The desire to complete the puzzle is so consuming they'll study her social media activity in search of a new puzzle piece.

In the meantime, they'll only be able to talk about the current aspect of their puzzle, which changes often.

Today you ask a boy: "Does she love you?" and he'll say "yes," because she has touched him on his shoulder while they were talking. Tomorrow you'll ask him the same question and you'll receive a different answer because she didn't even say "hi" to him this morning.

A boy in love lives in a state of constant reflection and contemplation.

Why?

Because he wants to know. He wants to be sure. He wants to predict what's going to happen next, so he can feel safe.

Both the autistic and the neurotypical boy lack an area in their brains specialized in interpreting in real-time if a girl loves them back or not.

Hence, they need to acquire as many bits of information about the girl as they can. Next, they evaluate them for a long as they're able to, by using Google and considering other people's opinion. They draw their conclusions. Next, they have to test these hypotheses whether they want it or not, in each new interaction with the girl.

Can you empathize with the boy's desire to know the truth? Can you feel his need to be alone in his bedroom and contemplate all the intricacies of the dating process? Can you recall how infatuation feels like and how much it hurts being forced to stop thinking about your love interest just so you can deal with the mundane tasks life keeps throwing at you throughout the day? Do you remember how much you wished to be able to stop whatever you were doing and let yourself be lost in your thoughts, wondering about your love interest?

Well, that's how the autistic brain feels about everything.

Take a moment to digest this last word, "everything."

Maybe you've heard the autistic brain lives in a constant state of contemplation. Maybe you've wondered what this meant. Now you know.

You also understand why downtime is so important for the autistic brain.

If someone with autism finds himself in a new situation, he'll need to process it through to understand it. He'll need to compare all that has happened with what he thought he knew about reality. Does this new experience fit in is worldview? If it doesn't he needs to tear his picture of reality apart and build a new one.

Everyone goes through this process when dealing with a new situation with unexpected results. This happens once in a while. Maybe if you are visiting a country with a completely different culture. But, for the most part, reality works more or less as expected by the neurotypical brain. There are surprises, but they fall within what you know reality can throw at you. However, for the autistic brain things are much different.

Due to the difficulties in processing emotional, social and abstract information, the autistic brain finds himself witnessing many unexpected outcomes. Without the ability to process social interactions trough dedicated neural networks, each new human interaction is as surprising as each new encounter with a person of a completely different culture.

This is just one of the reasons why the autistic brain needs frequent periods away from new information. This provides the brain with a precious resource: time to process new data and draw conclusions.

This also means that it's normal for an autistic person to change his mind about a subject whenever new data comes up. This shouldn't be interpreted as instability but as evidence of the intense desire to live in a way that is consistent with what he believes to be true and to speak with conviction about it.

This means that when the autistic needs space and time to process information, acquiring that silence and that time is as vital as drinking water when thirsty.

The empathy of others and good advice from mature people can help him process the information, but then he needs to be left alone. Nothing replaces being by himself, preferably listening to enjoyable music or doing stimming.

Sometimes the puzzle is too hard to figure out. Maybe reality has shown its ugly head too hard. Suffering bullying, going through a loss or enduring any other form of trauma can be too much to deal with.

If your boy or girl can't neutralize distressing thoughts he, or she, needs therapy, with cognitive therapy being recommended.

In simple terms, cognitive therapy consists of writing down what you are thinking about and evaluating it, also in writing. You draw a line in the middle of a piece of blank paper and write down the data you have for and against the truthfulness of each of your distressing thoughts.

Cognitive therapy also consists of learning many techniques. Some help the person to understand that emotions exist in varying degrees. The world is rarely either black or white. Others involve adjusting your viewpoint trough mental exercises such as examining a situation from several angles.

Some autistic people, whether by chance or by research or advice from others, develop their own ways of dealing with distressing thoughts.

Chapter 4, in this book, is an example of a method someone with autism can use to process social and emotional information faster.

When someone with autism is forced to describe the incomplete picture of the puzzle present in their mind, the result may be a condition called mutism. Mutism happens when the autistic is unable to transform the ideas and images inside his mind into a speakable language. He wants to talk but his mental translator is offline.

We can imagine words as cars stuck in traffic. No matter how fast those people desire to get out of there, they'll have to wait until the traffic jam dissipates. Then, the cars, slowly, we'll start to move again.

The same thing happens in mutism. We can imagine mutism as a kind of meltdown. Continuing to force an autistic person to communicate when he is suffering from mutism is an effective way to cause a meltdown even more severe or even a complete shutdown.

A shutdown happens when the autistic brain takes a "medical leave" and stops working, no matter how much the person wants it to. We can imagine this event as a defense mechanism, a kind of moderate vasovagal syndrome.

Sudden mutism and withdrawal are one of the reasons for the social phobia that often afflicts people with more moderate forms of autism.

When a person with autism is suffering from a mutism attack, this is a clear indication that he needs to be left alone in his world. Then, he's expected to recover.

If this recovery doesn't occur within the space of a day, some kind of "therapeutic" intervention is needed, such as the comfort given by the presence of a favorite person. If this kind of intervention fails, you might need the help of a health professional well acquainted with autism.

But please, remember to keep any psychologists or psychiatrists who are not well familiarized with autism as far away from your child as you can. This will avoid much suffering. The last thing you need is an over-medicated kid, or to receive advice indicating that you should be forcing the autistic child to behave like a neurotypical.

B. Understanding the Need for Controlling Emotions

The regular strategies someone with autism uses to exercise control over his emotions are (1) stimming, (2) the detailed processing of the information contributing to the emotional imbalance, and (3) the distraction obtained from devoting oneself to an obsession, like a hobby or a favorite person.

When I say "obsession," I don't mean it in a derogatory sense, but as an indication of the autistic ability to completely abstract himself from everything else while he is engaged in researching, reading, or interacting with something he just loves too much.

These special affections may involve trains, astronomy, math, board games, collection cards, Star Wars, an animal, construction blocks, a person, a book, a video game, an instrument, a physical activity, or whatever else you can think of.

Not all these obsessions are healthy though. For example, if your child devotes his time and energy to a person and then this person fails to reciprocate, this will be devastating. However, devoting his time and energy to astronomy or another field of science will make him — and the favorite person who listens to his explanations — a "little teacher" on the subject, as Hans Asperger once said.

In any case, these special interests will vary greatly depending on other factors, such as the degree of autism, sensory hypersensitivities, and the intellectual and emotional development of the autistic person.

In any case, there isn't much capacity for direct control over emotions without first receiving an emotional re-education, where emotional intelligence is taught in a concrete way compatible with the special interests of the autistic person.

This re-education exploits neuroplasticity, the brain's extraordinary ability to modify itself. Meaning we'll be using the brain areas that do work, such as those related to concrete thinking, and teach them to take on the work of the areas that aren't working properly, such as those related to emotional processing.

Moreover, since understanding what one is feeling is difficult for someone with autism, the empathy of others, and the security of knowing that such support is always available, is vital.

Finally, the expression of sentiments through writing, photography, plastic arts or theater is another way of exercising some control over emotions.

The right music at the right time also has a very immediate and powerful effect on emotions.

We all have the need to control our emotional impulses and stress levels. A person with autism is no exception. It's just that the strategies must be different, adapted to the atypical neurological configuration of the autistic brain.

C. The Need to Protect Oneself from Sensory Hypersensitivities

Many autistic individuals have several sensory hypersensitivities. These are caused by the way their brain deals with information and not by a dysfunction in the sensory organs. It's as if their brain either greatly amplified, or decreased, the signal it's receiving.

If a hypersensitivity relates to noise levels it's necessary to cover one's ears, but if the hypersensitivity is visual it may be necessary to close one's eyes or move to a place with less visual information; somewhere without so many people moving around or without so many colorful patterns.

Clothes with scratching labels, itching fabrics or that are uncomfortable in some other way, will also cause much distress to someone with autism.

The impact of a friendly slap to the back can be quite uncomfortable, even causing pain. In the same way, a handshake that turns into a hand squeezing war may get you blacklisted by the person with autism.

Strong smells, the noise produced by a motorcycle engine, flickering lights — that sometimes only the autistic person has enough sensitivity to detect, like the flickering produced by fluorescent light bulbs — will all gradually lead to sensory overload and a subsequent meltdown.

Specific strategies and a detailed analysis of each of the main senses are available in Chapter 6.

D. The Need to Rest

Adrenaline and the bodily transformations it promotes are very exhausting.

This wear and tear is at the origin of many depressions.

In the case of the autistic individual, besides all the other sources of stress universal to humans, there are some extra ones, specific to autism:

- Having to process new information while under pressure. This would be distracting and relaxing to a neurotypical person but can be a source of exhaustion for someone with autism.

- Dealing with people outside of his circle of favorite people.

- Having a sensory hypersensitivity stimulated by the environment.

In and of itself, stress wears you down.

In addition, stress makes it harder to relax and fall asleep. It sabotages the natural strategies our body uses to recover its mental and physical energy.

Moreover, stress damages the digestive system in many ways. It affects the appetite and the quality of the intestinal flora. In turn, this reduces the person's ability to absorb the nutrients present in the food being eaten.

Extra rest is therefore vital. Resting prevents some meltdowns and, when they do occur, resting enhances recovery.

At this point, you can probably understand that getting up every day and trying to lead a normal life, "pretending to be normal," can be quite a heroic act for someone with a level of autism that allows him to work or attend school.

The need to be alone and rest after a social interaction is as real as the need to stop and breath after running a marathon. It's as real as the need to rest after spending an hour solving complex mathematical problems. This need is entirely biological and inescapable.

Pushing the autistic to make a decision when he needs to process information or rest is akin to forcing the panting marathoner to sing. And it can lead to a meltdown.

E. The Need for Support

People with autism are not antisocial or anti-people. They simply tend to feel a lot of stress when they are around others. This happens because they have a hard time understanding people and avoiding bullying and intimidation.

The truth is that it's easy for someone with autism to become a favorite victim of bullies.

He walks in a strange way, thinks and speaks in an unusual, often pompous, manner. His interests are very narrow and he's often alone. It's the perfect target.

The same strangeness holds true for a girl with autism. Except this girl will have the tendency to hang out with the boys who might look at her unusual behavior as girly.

Even when loving people try to help someone with autism, they try to do it in the language of neurotypicals. Perhaps encouraging the person to avoid stimming or to simply "let go" of his meltdowns and sensory hypersensitivities.

Even other people with autism may be unable to provide the necessary support. Imagine an autistic person who is sensitive to noise spending time with one who loves listening to loud music.

In this way, real support can only come from someone who understands autism at a deeper level. This type of support will help meet the other special needs referred here and will make survival a much easier ordeal.

Family, employers, teachers and educators, anyone who deals daily with an autistic, needs to understand the biological functions of stimming and meltdowns.

This will allow them to provide the necessary support when a meltdown is about to occur.

They can do this by (1) giving the necessary empathy — especially in the case of a meltdown primarily caused by distressing thoughts, (2) helping the person protect himself from disturbing sensory stimuli — in the case of a meltdown due to sensory overload, and (3) removing the person from a crowded place.

When in the presence of people, the autistic brain is compelled to continually process "what is the right thing to say next" and "what is the right thing to do next." This is especially true when in the presence of people with whom he's not well acquainted.

What if this support fails to prevent a meltdown?

If a meltdown does occur, it's important to remind the autistic person that a meltdown is just the natural, and uncontrollable, reaction from his nervous system to the wear and tear it underwent. A meltdown doesn't reveal anything at all about the person's character, nor is it indicative of neurological problems, nor does it cause such problems. It's only a normal and inevitable physiological process in the autistic whenever their nervous system is overwhelmed.

At best, the person can do choose to cry instead of becoming violent, but apart from that, there isn't much else he can do.

This kind of informed support is of special importance immediately before, during and right after a meltdown.

You, my reader, have in your possession the information necessary to become that kind of person for any autistic. However, the more information you seek to acquire, either through the scientific literature or through the reading of biographical works, the better.

Use this information to provide support. Use it to educate others on how to help. Be sure to make use of what you have learned here.

Chapter 10

The Difficulties of Receiving an Official Diagnosis

An official diagnosis is important because people with autism are sensitive to medications. For example, in the case of antidepressants, Temple Grandin advises someone with autism to start with ⅓ (33%) of the recommended dose. In the case of other drugs, it is necessary to consider that the recommended dose for someone with autism can be from ¼ (25%) to ½ (50%) of the dose used with other people without autism.

Otherwise, the autistic person may end up suffering more side effects than normal. This may cause some doctors to regard the person as a hypochondriac, leading the person to become afraid of medications and physicians.

The less visible the underlying autism the harder it'll be to get diagnosed. People with Asperger's syndrome can go through life without ever receiving the correct diagnosis.

If this person ends up with depression and seeks psychiatric help from a doctor unfamiliar with autism, he may end up being misdiagnosed with some kind of mental illnesses requiring strong medication.

What's the result?

You will see autistic patients being treated with powerful tranquilizers or unnecessary antipsychotics. This will only increase the suffering and the effects of these medications on the nervous system will only mask even more the underlying autism.

Illnesses that are often confused with some particularities of autism

Are you unsure if you have autism? Here's a non-exhaustive list of conditions that can be misdiagnosed by a health professional unfamiliar with autism.

- The difficulty to ignore intrusive sensory stimuli and the anxiety of feeling something unknown in the body can be regarded as an indication of hypochondria. Add to this the heightened sensitivity to medications, and it's easy to understand why a doctor could ignore a patient's complaints and go for a **hypochondria** diagnosis.

- The need to follow routines, and to organize things in a way that reduces the need to process new information, can be isolated from the other symptoms of autism, and result in a diagnosis of **Obsessive-Compulsion Disorder.**

- The mood swings generated as information is processed can be interpreted as emotional instability. Coupled with meltdowns, which would be interpreted as regular nervous breakdowns, all this apparent emotional volatility could lead to a misdiagnosis of **Borderline Personality Disorder**.

- Since the autistic child is unable to adequately contain the euphoria he feels when involved in a project he loves, he's able to go on without food or sleep. This can be confused with the manic phase of bipolarity. In turn, depressive meltdowns would be regarded as the depressive phase of bipolarity. Leading to the misdiagnosis of **Bipolar Disorder**.

- When an autistic person interacts with others, he easily acquires their mannerisms and accent, as well as copying their facial expressions. Coupled with his contemplative personality and the continual search for the answer to the question "who am I?" a more audacious health professional may risk a diagnosis of **Dissociative Identity Disorder** or another equally exotic mental illness.

- When an autistic person isolates himself because of his social interaction difficulties, his creative mind can end up develop detailed worlds and stories, including imaginary friends, which can lead to the misdiagnosis of **Schizophrenia**.

- A meltdown of depressive nature along with the subsequent withdrawal period may be confused with **Major Depression**.

- The ever-present anxiety can be mistakenly analyzed in isolation from the other symptoms of autism. That way, the doctor may think that it all boils down to some sort of **phobia** or an **anxiety disorder**. Following this isolated diagnosis, stronger anxiolytics may end up being prescribed.

- Stimming can be misdiagnosed as **hyperactivity**. Because of this, the vital role of stimming as an external regulator of emotions would be ignored. The doctor would identify stimming as a behavior to be suppressed.

- The brain's struggles to ignore new sensory stimuli may lead the autistic to give the appearance of someone who suffers from **Attention Deficit Disorder.**

- Because of his difficulties in generating empathy intuitively and due to the problems in the field of theory of mind, someone with autism attempts to empathize by looking inside himself in search for personal experiences similar to the situation he's trying to empathize with. This allows him to gain a deeper understanding of what the other person might be feeling. Because of this internal process, the autistic person tends to talk a lot about himself, instead of focusing his attention on the other person. This can lead to a misdiagnosis of **Narcissistic Personality Disorder**.

Of course, these diseases can, and sometimes do occur along with autism, as the autistic person isn't immune to them.

However, if you or your child were diagnosed with any of these mental illnesses, before embarking on a journey of medication, it's important to verify if the problem isn't in the daily routine.

After all, a routine that prevents the autistic from using the appropriate strategies to meet his special needs may give rise to symptoms that mimic serious mental illnesses, when in fact it's just the autism.

For example, if in his daily routine the autistic is always in the company of other people, this will greatly increase the need to stim, the frequency and intensity of his meltdowns and the need for him to remain isolated with his obsessions late into the night.

So, what's going on?

Should he be diagnosed as bipolar or borderline and medicated accordingly? No. He just needs to adjust his routine a bit, creating more opportunities to be alone after each demanding social interaction so he can restore his mental energy.

Likewise, if parents are forbidding the autistic child from stimming and the child's behavior and meltdowns keep worsening, does it make sense to diagnose the child with attention deficit disorder and drug him? Certainly not.

However, therapies that help the autistic person attend to the root of their problems are always helpful. These include therapies that teach him strategies for dealing with distressing thoughts, such as cognitive therapy, or exercises that increase his emotional intelligence — like those presented in Chapter 4.

Chapter 11

A New Vocabulary

In this book, we have used many words and phrases you may not have been familiar with. But what if they became common? At home, in the classroom, and in the workplace?

Before the teacher would tell parents:

1. Your child has many difficulties in understanding what we teach him.

2. He has numerous challenges expressing empathy.

3. He is very agitated, we don't know what else to do.

4. Your kid keeps having anger outbursts.

5. He always seems to be lost in her own world.

But with the new vocabulary the teacher would say:

1. We have adapted our teaching methods to better suit your child's unique learning style. We now include many examples using a clear, concise and concrete language. We can already see an increase in his interest and his grades are beginning to reflect that.

2. We have used these same teaching techniques to teach him about emotional intelligence and the simple strategies he can implement to improve his ability to communicate with others. We have noticed significant improvements.

3. This week, we noticed that your son was stimming more than usual. So, we asked you to meet with us so that we can do a joint evaluation of your child's daily routine, to see if any element can be rearranged to take into account his special needs.

4. Today your son had several meltdowns. So, we recommend you take him home for the rest of the afternoon. He needs some alone time, so he can rest and

recover. Tomorrow, if he's doing better, we'd love to have him back with us.

5. We have learned to ask many questions about his special interests. It's true that sometimes he'll answer with a lengthy explanation, but we've noticed how he stays engaged. He treats us as if you had his age. Seeing him so interested in communicating with us is so gratifying.

Before the father or the mother would think:

1. Why won't my daughter stay still for a moment? Should I try to stop her and punish her for doing this all the time?

2. I don't know what else to do! The relapses are becoming more and more frequent and uncontrollable, I fear that my son will end up in a psychiatric hospital.

3. It seems my son doesn't care about my feelings. He doesn't even know I exist.

4. How can she be always tired? Why doesn't she help me more? What a lazy child.

5. Why does he always have to make a scene in the supermarket?

But with the new vocabulary they would think:

1. She keeps stimming. First, I must do some detective work and try to figure out what sensory stimuli may be stressing her out. Next, I need to reevaluate her daily routine and see if I can reduce the total amount of interaction time she's having with other people, so she can have more time to recover her mental energy. Finally, I must try to find out if there is anything that is troubling her or if her stimming is a sign of pain or of another kind of physical discomfort.

2. My son keeps having meltdowns and I don't know what else to do. I need to seek medical help from a health

professional who is well acquainted with autism so that my child doesn't end up unnecessarily medicated or institutionalized in a place where their sensory sensitivities would hardly be taken into consideration.

3. I need to understand what topics fascinate my son and learn about them. I need to educate him about emotional intelligence using his obsessions as a for my examples. I need to remember to use a direct and concrete teaching style as much as possible.

4. My daughter is getting tired increasingly fast. This is a sign that her body is frequently activating the stress response. I need to examine her daily routine and find what's triggering all this stress. Until then, I will let our house be her refuge.

5. A supermarket is a place with lots of unknown people and with a large number of sensory stimuli. I don't want my son to always stay at home when I go shopping, but I don't want him to stay in the supermarket until he has exhausted all his mental energy. I will try to be more balanced and reduce the total time I spend with him in the supermarket. I'm going to use his stimming to gauge when it's time to go home. That way, he won't develop an aversion to supermarkets. As long as I keep respecting his limits I'm sure he will desensitize over time, and his tolerance for supermarkets will increase.

In addition, the very way the autistic person communicates — if he has that capacity — with his parents, teachers, and employers can change.

Before he would simply isolate himself, stimming. He would have meltdowns and be left wondering what's wrong with him. But now he can start using the new vocabulary to help others understand him better. For example, instead of expecting others to try to figure out how close he is to a meltdown, he might simply inform them.

This new way of thinking changes the entire paradigm of autism.

We no longer look at the diagnosis but at each individual symptom and the special needs that this symptom is revealing.

Then, appropriate strategies can be used to meet those needs. In the end, everyone wins.

Chapter 12

Why Can We Have Hope for Improvement?

Depression has been called "the curse of the strong." Why? For example, imagine having to care for an old parent with Alzheimer's while having a full-time job and two children of your own. Would you quit? Not if you're strong.

A strong person will tend to hold on to the challenge. Even to the point of emotional exhaustion.

At this point, others would've thrown in the towel and give up, but not the mighty one. These people choose to hold on until their emotional system can't endure it any longer. Then, they'll develop clinical depression. And still, they won't quit.

Why? Where are they drawing their strength from?

From their love for their parents.

Could this same strength be present in someone with autism?

Yes. Their inner power is indisputable, for it allows them to get up each day despite their struggles.

In the case of the Asperger, for example, author Rudy Simone mentioned that the reason why these people — especially women — are so compassionate and gentle is due to all the hardships they had to endure.

These hardships, however, take their toll.

A recipe for compassion

Throughout their lives, those on the spectrum have gone through immeasurable amounts of emotional distress along with misdiagnoses, labels, bullying, and incomprehension from those around them. Because of this, autistic people know what it's like to suffer and they avoid saying or doing something that causes suffering to others.

Unfortunately, they also have to deal with meltdowns, major difficulties in expressing empathy and exercising self-control, and the near-constant emotional distress.

It's easy to imagine why someone with autism tends to develop self-esteem problems. How can you help?

The next step

Because of all their internal strength, we can expect that with the help of knowledgeable parents and educators, small but key adjustments in their daily routines can cause significant changes in their quality of life.

Practical applications

One of the books by Tony Attwood, the acclaimed autism researcher, has the following quote from someone with Asperger, who said to him:

« We don't have emotional skin or protection. We are exposed, and that is why we hide. »

This means that if he's very enthusiastic about a project, although he can spend an entire day working on it, a very negative comment from another person can be enough to make him abandon it. Why? Because he'll feel sad and disappointed, unable to reconcile these negative emotions with his previous enthusiasm. Moreover, he would be annoyed at the person who, from his perspective, took away his enthusiasm.

Autistics, especially those with Asperger's syndrome, place their sense of identity in the things they do. This means that when someone criticizes their work they feel it as if they were the ones being criticized.

As an individual with autism said:

« Criticism [related to an ongoing project] really hurts. I only feel better after going home and analyzing everything that has been said to me, sometimes for days on end. »

On the other hand, autistic people are very sensitive to praise. Even a small compliment can be enough to leave them with a lasting feeling of joy.

The take home point?

Your words have a tremendous power over the autistic person. Use them to motivate the person to overcome his struggles.

One your child or student with deep autism learns to recognize a new word praise him as if he had learned to speak a whole new language. From his perspective, it was such a big of a victory.

Thousands, perhaps millions, of neural networks had to reorganize themselves in ways that brain had never even imagine. All this, just so he could recognize one word.

His mind wasn't built for language, but now that he has learned to recognize one word nothing is stopping him from learning another.

If you're dealing with Asperger praise every step towards greater emotional intelligence. Can he now distinguish between shades of sadness in others' facial expressions? Fantastic. That's a feat for the autistic brain. Celebrate it and praise it accordingly.

Never forget how special their needs are

Every autistic person is different in how they deal with reality, choose to stim, and in how they express their eternally unfinished puzzle with the world. But I believe that everyone on the autism spectrum has the special needs I have described in common.

These needs, natural to mankind, require specific strategies you must be aware of.

This awareness must be present at all names. Write them down if must: Both the needs and the special strategies to meet them.

Are you on the spectrum too?

Statistically, if a family member has autism, it's likely that the more immediate members will also have some of the traits, even to the point of being diagnosed too, because of the genetic factors.

Many adults only discover that they have more moderate forms of autism, such as Asperger's, later in life, when one of their own children is diagnosed.

Furthermore, given the rather specific personality of an autistic person, it's likely that his closest friends — the favorite people with whom he feels almost no mental wear and tear — also have such traits.

Don't believe everything you read on the Internet about autism

Sometimes, the information freely available on the Internet about autism can become depressing. Why? Because you'll learn about the struggles of bloggers and YouTubers with autism, who don't know how to address their special needs. These men and women don't have people like you around them. They've yet to meet someone educated on autism.

However, this helps us understand what it is like to live with autism when you don't have access to the right support.

This should motivate each one of us to recognize the value of what you've learned and the need to share it with other autistic people and their families and educators.

After all, if someone has a moderate form of autism and never learns to use the right strategies to meet his special needs, what will become of his life?

Living with Autism without knowing about It

We can imagine why someone who doesn't know he's on the spectrum would end up developing a daily routine that doesn't take his autism into consideration. He'll be unable to adjust his life to account for his special needs.

Add to this the many bad life-changing decisions, depression, overmedication, and the despair of living without really knowing oneself.

The freedom that comes from knowing

In conclusion, note these elucidating words:

> « Knowing that I have Asperger has made me forgive myself for many things that have happened in my past, gave me a greater understanding about who I am, and allowed me to begin to change the way I interact with the world to avoid the meltdowns and the other things caused by Asperger. »

Whether or not you are the one with autism, please use the information contained in this book to obtain a greater control over your own life and the life of those with autism around you. This will increase your quality of life and give you the joy of contributing to someone else's well-being.

And, so you can really grasp what can be accomplished when autism is under control, look at the biographies of some of these people:

- Mozart

- Nikola Tesla

- Thomas Jefferson

- Albert Einstein

- Ludwig Wittgenstein

These men are believed by some experts to have had moderate forms of autism. Not that they could have been diagnosed at a time when autism was unknown, but their life and work revealed many of the characteristics that we now associate with autism.

This shows us the intellectual and artistic capacity latent in the same brain that has such a great difficulty in dealing with routine changes, loud noises or even expressing empathy.

Is there hope?

Some, perhaps with too much enthusiasm, even claim that people with Asperger's are responsible for the intellectual advancement in the world.

In some cases, having Asperger's really means having an intellect with special abilities, including the capacity to acquire university-level knowledge about a topic within months, learning a language with ease, art creation or even identifying patterns and links where no one else can see them. I've yet to meet someone with Asperger's without some kind of gift, even if it's an encyclopedic knowledge of Pokémon.

In the case of classical autism, cases such as that of Temple Grandin and Rain K. Kaufman demonstrate that even the deep autistic can recover to the point of leading a satisfactory and successful life.

So, the answer is: Yes, there is hope.

Autism is considered a developmental disorder. In this case, neural plasticity explains why even someone with deep autism has the potential to gain some degree of control over his impulses, knowledge about his emotions or the ability to interact socially.

After all, can't a thin person build up his physique?

Then, why shouldn't someone with autism be able to develop the ability to interpret social information?

Over time, through repetition and the introduction of new experiences, someone with autism will possess a sufficiently large base of concrete examples that he'll be able to understand how to deal with entirely new social situations.

However, just as a person genetically predisposed to being thin has a harder time gaining much muscle, so does the autistic brain face more challenges to develop social skills.

Someone with autism may never develop the same level of social aptitude as someone whose brain was born with all the necessary machinery. But this is very different from the widespread concept, present in the movies and in the media, that having autism is the end of the line and that there is nothing one can do about it.

Besides, normal is boring. Don't you agree?

Without autism, how would we have all the inventions of Nikola Tesla? Or the scientific advances idealized by Albert Einstein or computers and the Internet? Truth be told, many of today's computer geniuses have many of the signs of moderate autism.

I conclude by inviting the reader to take a closer look at the appendix that follows. In it, you'll find four supplements that relieved the symptoms of autism, as described in published scientific studies.

Appendix

Four supplements that relieved the symptoms of autism in published scientific studies

Although the following statements don't replace the need for a consultation with a doctor, they do show us that there's always something that can be done to help a person with autism, even when everyone else tells you otherwise.

In each case, references to the specific clinical studies are provided. These can be given to your doctor or to anyone else who may wish to analyze them.

Vitamin D3

As we have noted, while there are many theories about the many possible causes of autism, there's no agreement between experts. However, in recent times, scientists have discovered something extraordinary: the relationship between vitamin D and autism.

The first point is that if you have autism, vitamin D supplementation has a good potential to improve your symptoms.[5] Especially when you surpass the 40 ng/mL mark.[6] In addition, it seems that the sooner you begin supplementing, the greater the benefit.[7]

What's more, recent research demonstrates that a **woman's vitamin D level during pregnancy is directly related to her baby's chances of developing an autistic brain**.[8, 9, 10]

In addition, there is evidence of a relationship between vitamin D deficiency and the development of alexithymia — the name given to the inability to identify and describe the emotions you are feeling — one of the hallmarks of autism.[11]

So, if you, or someone you know, is pregnant or plans to become pregnant it's vital that you get to know your vitamin D levels and the benefits of vitamin D supplementation. But, of course, always

---

[5]Jia F, Wang B, Shan L, Xu Z, Staal WG, Du L. Core symptoms of autism improved after vitamin D supplementation. Pediatrics. 2015;135(1):e196-8. https://www.ncbi.nlm.nih.gov/pubmed/25511123

[6]Saad K, Abdel-rahman AA, Elserogy YM, et al. Vitamin D status in autism spectrum disorders and the efficacy of vitamin D supplementation in autistic children. Nutr Neurosci. 2016;19(8):346-351.https://www.ncbi.nlm.nih.gov/pubmed/25876214

[7]Feng J, Shan L, Du L, et al. Clinical improvement following vitamin D3 supplementation in Autism Spectrum Disorder. Nutr Neurosci. 2016; https://www.ncbi.nlm.nih.gov/pubmed/26783092

[8]Cannell JJ. Vitamin D and autism, what's new?. Rev Endocr Metab Disord. 2017;18(2):183-193. https://www.ncbi.nlm.nih.gov/pubmed/28217829

[9]Cannell JJ, Grant WB. What is the role of vitamin D in autism?. Dermatoendocrinol. 2013;5(1):199-204. https://www.ncbi.nlm.nih.gov/pubmed/24494055

[10]Duan XY, Jia FY, Jiang HY. [Relationship between vitamin D and autism spectrum disorder]. Zhongguo Dang Dai Er Ke Za Zhi. 2013;15(8):698-702. https://www.ncbi.nlm.nih.gov/pubmed/23965890

[11]Altbäcker A, Plózer E, Darnai G, et al. Alexithymia is associated with low level of vitamin D in young healthy adults. Nutr Neurosci. 2014;17(6):284-8. https://www.ncbi.nlm.nih.gov/pubmed/24593042

under proper medical supervision, given the fragility of the developing fetus.

Currently, autism, either moderate or profound, affects 1 in 68 people. With boys being 4 times more affected than girls.[12]

Hence, in my book on safe supplementation with high doses of vitamin D, we raised this question: "How would these statistics change if all mothers supplemented with an appropriate level of vitamin D during pregnancy?"

The adequate blood test to check our vitamin levels D is the one that verifies the levels of **Cholecalciferol** or **25(OH)D3**. Other names for this test include "Calcifediol", "Calcidiol", "25(OH)D" and "25-hydroxycholecalciferol."

The reference values according to the Brazilian Society of Clinical Pathology and the Brazilian Society of Endocrinology and Metabolism are as follows:

- Above 20 ng/mL is the desired value.

- Between 30 and 60 ng/mL is the recommended value for groups at risk like the elderly, pregnant women, infants, patients with rickets/osteomalacia, osteoporosis, patients with a history of falls and fractures, secondary causes of osteoporosis (diseases and medications), hyperparathyroidism, inflammatory diseases, autoimmune diseases, chronic kidney disease and malabsorption syndromes (clinical or post-surgical).

- Above 100 ng/mL carries the risk of toxicity and hypercalcemia.[13]

In any case, the daily dose of vitamin D considered safe **for adults** is 10,000 international units (IU). This dosage is much higher than the recommended daily allowance (RDA) of 600 IU for premenopausal women.

People with difficulties in vitamin D metabolism require doses **much higher than 600 IU in order** to obtain an adequate therapeutic effect. However, several safety procedures need to be

---

[12] https://www.ncbi.nlm.nih.gov/pubmedhealth/PMHT0024869/

[13] http://www.sbpc.org.br/noticias-e-comunicacao/novos-intervalos-de-referencia-de-vitamina-d/

followed to ensure that these high doses won't cause serious problems.

These procedures are discussed in detail in my book on Vitamin D and Vitamin K2 and include testing one's blood and 24-hour urine calcium levels and parathyroid hormone (PTH) levels, dietary calcium restrictions, the ingestion of vitamin D co-factors, such as vitamin K2, magnesium and vitamin B2 and the consumption of high amounts of liquids, on the order of 2.5 liters (2.64 quarts) per day.

The administration of any supplement during pregnancy, or to a child, should only be done after checking with a qualified doctor that this can be done safely.

With this in mind, we can now dig deeper into this subject.

In one of the studies involving women who already had at least one child with autism, the following vitamin D dosages were used:

- 5,000 IU daily during gestation, this dose being in most cases initiated only from the second quarter.

- 7,000 IU per day throughout the entire breastfeeding period. (Note that these 7,000 IU were taken daily by the mother, not by the child).

- If the child stopped drinking the mother's milk, she (the child) would start supplementation with 1,000 IU daily until she was 3 years old.

For example, if the child suckled up to the age of 12 months, that would mean the child would start taking 1,000 IU of vitamin D from that point on and up to the age of 36 months.

After that period, researchers looked at the percentage of children who eventually developed autism. Then, they looked at the probability of these women having an autistic child — remember these are women who already had at least one autistic child.

What was the conclusion?

When a woman who has had a child with autism has another child, there's a 20 percent chance that this new child will develop autism. However, only 5% of the children involved in the study developed autism. That is, of the 19 children involved, only 1 eventually developed autism.[14]

This was a study of small proportions, but it illustrates the potential of vitamin D when administered to the mother during pregnancy and breastfeeding period and to the child after this breastfeeding period ends and up until the age of 36 months.

In another study,[15] 106 children with autism who had blood levels of vitamin D below 30 ng/mL received a daily dose of vitamin D corresponding to 300 IU for each kilogram of body mass (300 IU per 2.20 pounds), but without ever exceeding daily 5,000 IU. 83 children completed 3 months of treatment.

What was the result?

67 of the 83 children who received vitamin D showed improvement in their autistic symptoms.

Why should there be a relationship between vitamin D and autism?

Dr. John J. Cannel from the Vitamin D Council,[16] in one of his papers published in the journal *Medical Hypothesis*,[17] presents some arguments difficult to ignore:

- "The apparent increase in the prevalence of autism over the last 20 years [between 1987 and 2007, when Dr. Cannel published his work] corresponds with increasing medical advice to avoid the sun, advice that has probably lowered vitamin D levels and would theoretically greatly lower activated vitamin D (calcitriol) levels in developing brains."

- "Animal data has repeatedly shown that severe vitamin D

---

[14]Stubbs G, Henley K, Green J. Autism: Will vitamin D supplementation during pregnancy and early childhood reduces the recurrence rate of autism in newborn siblings ?. Med Hypotheses. 2016; 88: 74-8.
https://www.ncbi.nlm.nih.gov/pubmed/26880644

[15]Saad K, Abdel-Rahman AA, Elserogy YM, et al. Vitamin D status in autism spectrum disorders and the efficacy of vitamin D supplementation in autistic children. Nutr Neurosci. 2016: 19 (8): 346-351.
https://www.ncbi.nlm.nih.gov/pubmed/25876214

[16]Link: www.vitamindcouncil.org

[17]Cannell JJ. Autism and vitamin D. Med Hypotheses. 2008; 70 (4): 750-9.
https://www.ncbi.nlm.nih.gov/pubmed/17920208

deficiency during gestation dysregulates dozens of proteins involved in brain development and leads to rat pups with increased brain size and enlarged ventricles, abnormalities similar to those found in autistic children."

- "Children with the Williams Syndrome, who can have greatly elevated calcitriol [activated vitamin D] levels in early infancy, usually have phenotypes [or characteristics] that are the opposite of autism."

- "Children with vitamin D deficient rickets have several autistic markers that apparently disappear with high-dose vitamin D treatment."

- "Estrogen and testosterone have very different effects on calcitriol's metabolism, differences that may explain the striking male/female sex ratios in autism."

- "Calcitriol down-regulates production of inflammatory cytokines in the brain, cytokines that have been associated with autism."

- "Consumption of vitamin D containing fish during pregnancy reduces autistic symptoms in offspring."

- "Autism is more common in areas of impaired UVB [ultraviolet B radiation, the kind of solar radiation involved in the metabolism of vitamin D] penetration such as poleward latitudes, urban areas, areas with high air pollution, and areas of high precipitation. [this because the cloudy or rainy weather blocks UVB radiation]."

- "Autism is more common in dark-skinned persons and severe maternal vitamin D deficiency is exceptionally common [in] the dark-skinned."

In addition, in another paper published in the same journal, Dr. Cannel talks about how summer seems associated with a reduction in the symptoms of autism in some children, evidencing a potential relationship between the production of vitamin D and the symptoms of autism.[18]

Something like this wouldn't be surprising because of the intimate relationship between vitamin D and brain development and between vitamin D and several other processes involved in autism like the activation and regulation of the stress response.[19]

In any case, the cause of autism is still a topic with many uncertainties and involved in much debate. What practical nuggets of wisdom can we extract from this hypothesis?

Let us see:

1. Supplementing the mother with adequate doses of vitamin D during pregnancy and breastfeeding may benefit the mother and the baby, as long as there are no specific health problems that could put those benefits at risk, like hypercalcemia or a pre-existing renal impairment. These are two problems a regular panel of blood tests could rule out.

2. Supplementing the baby during the first years of his life plays a key role in the healthy development of the child's brain. Even if the child eventually develops autism, this autism is expected to be more moderate, since the effect of vitamin D on the brain involves increasing the body's ability to repair DNA, reducing inflammation, increasing the tolerance to convulsions, increasing the production of regulatory T lymphocytes, protecting the mitochondria responsible for producing cellular energy, and reducing oxidative stress by promoting the production of

---

[18] Cannell JJ. Autism, will vitamin D treat core symptoms ?. Med Hypotheses. 2013; 81 (2): 195-8. https://www.ncbi.nlm.nih.gov/pubmed/23725905

[19] Spedding S. Vitamin D and Depression: A Systematic Review and Meta-Analysis Comparing Studies with and without Biological Flaws. *Nutrients*. 2014; 6 (4): 1501-1518. doi: 10.3390 / nu6041501. https://www.ncbi.nlm.nih.gov/pmc/articles/PMC4011048/

glutathione.[20]

3. Adequate levels of vitamin D are beneficial to anyone, regardless of age or health.

The need to be careful about taking any drugs that affect the metabolism of vitamin D during pregnancy like antacids and cortisone and its derivatives.

---

[20] Cannell JJ. Autism and vitamin D. Med Hypotheses. 2008; 70 (4): 750-9. https://www.ncbi.nlm.nih.gov/pubmed/17920208

L-Carnitine

In one study, 100 mg of carnitine per kilogram of body weight were given daily to children with autism. This dose was taken for 6 months. What was the conclusion of the researchers? "L-carnitine therapy (100 mg/kg body weight/day) administered for 6 months significantly improved the autism severity, but subsequent studies are recommended."[21]

How do you calculate a dose of 100 mg/kg?

This means that you first convert the weight from pounds to **kilograms.** With each pound corresponding to 0.4535 kilograms of body mass. Next, you multiply the final number by 100 and you get the daily dose in milligrams

For example, a 45-pound child would end up taking roughly 2 grams of l-carnitine per day. This is because 45 pounds x 0.4535 x 100 mg equals nearly 2,041 mg.

For a child weighing 110 pounds, the daily dose would be 5 grams, since 110 pounds x 0.4535 x 100 mg = 4.988 mg, almost 5,000 mg.

Similar results were reported even at lower doses of **50 mg/kg/day** for a period of 3 months.[22] That is, half the dose used in the first study.

According to some researchers, a defect in the mitochondria of the cells is at the origin of the relationship between carnitine and autism.[23]

A deficiency in one of the genes responsible for controlling the functions involving carnitine and the mitochondria — the TMLHE gene[24] — has been pointed out as the reason for this relationship.

There was even at least one case described in the medical literature in which supplementation with carnitine was responsible

---

[21] https://www.sciencedirect.com/science/article/pii/S1750946712000827

[22] Geier DA, Kern JK, Davis G, et al. A prospective double-blind, randomized clinical trial of levocarnitine to treat autism spectrum disorders. Med Sci Monit. 2011;17(6):PI15-23. https://www.ncbi.nlm.nih.gov/pubmed/21629200

[23] Filipek PA, Juranek J, Nguyen MT, Cummings C, Gargus JJ. Relative carnitine deficiency in autism. J Autism Dev Disord. 2004;34(6):615-23. https://www.ncbi.nlm.nih.gov/pubmed/15679182

[24] http://www.genecards.org/cgi-bin/carddisp.pl?gene=TMLHE

for the recovery of a 4-year-old child who was beginning to exhibit the symptoms of autism.[25]

As for side effects, the administration of carnitine is advised against to those who **have had** convulsions. In addition, carnitine can worsen the symptoms of hypothyroidism — the name given to diseased and underactive thyroid gland.[26]

---

[25] Ziats MN, Comeaux MS, Yang Y, et al. Improvement of regressive autism symptoms in a child with TMLHE deficiency following carnitine supplementation. Am J Med Genet A. 2015;167A(9):2162-7.
https://www.ncbi.nlm.nih.gov/pubmed/25943046
[26] https://www.webmd.com/vitamins-supplements/ingredientmono-1026-l-carnitine.aspx?activeingredientid=1026&activeingredientname=l-carnitine

N-Acetylcysteine (NAC)

N-acetylcysteine (NAC) supplementation has been demonstrated to, specifically, improve the irritability resulting from autism.

This means that, in addition to stimming and the emotional intelligence strategies defined in chapter 4, NAC may become yet another tool available to help the autistic person cope with his emotions.[27]

The study in question lasted for 12 weeks.

During the first 4 weeks, the daily dose of NAC was of 900 mg. In the following 4 weeks, a dose of 900 mg was given twice per day — a total of 1,800 mg per day. In the last 4 weeks of the study, the dose of NAC was administered 3 times a day — a total of 2,700 mg per day.

	NAC	Total daily dose of NAC
Week 1 to 4	900 mg - once per day	900 mg/day
Week 5 to 8	900 mg — twice per day	1,800 mg/day
Week 9 to 12	900 mg - 3 times per day	2,700 mg/day

Some of the side effects observed in some study participants included constipation, diarrhea, nausea, and vomiting. Caution should, therefore, be exercised. This is one of the reasons researchers start with a lower dose.

The rationale behind the use of NAC has to do with a hypothesis linking oxidative stress and abnormalities in the glutamatergic pathways — that is, in the pathways related to glutamate, which is a neurotransmitter — with autism. Since NAC is a glutamatergic modulator and antioxidant, it was used in the study.

---

[27]Hardan AY, Fung LK, Libove RA, et al. A randomized controlled pilot trial of oral N-acetylcysteine in children with autism. Biol Psychiatry. 2012;71(11):956-61. https://www.ncbi.nlm.nih.gov/pubmed/22342106

Digestive Enzymes

Due to the link between the health of our digestive system and the proper functioning of the brain, several researchers have tried to determine what effect, if any, digestive enzymes supplementation could have on the symptoms of autism.[28]

During the 3-month study, significant improvements in emotional response and behavior were observed, as well as improvements in gastrointestinal symptoms.

The digestive enzymes used in the study were just two: **papain** and **pepsin**.

Each day, study participants received 15 ml of the liquid containing the enzymes. 5 ml before each of the three main meals.

This corresponds, according to the data provided by the study, to 80 milligrams of papain and 40 milligrams of pepsin per 5 ml.

	Papain	Pepsin
Before breakfast	80 mg	40 mg
Before lunch	80 mg	40 mg
Before dinner	80 mg	40 mg
Daily total:	240 mg	120 mg

The reported side effects were mild and included some cases of rash, itching and abdominal pain.

---

[28]Saad K, Eltayeb AA, Mohamad IL, et al. A Randomized, Placebo-controlled Trial of Digestive Enzymes in Children with Autism Spectrum Disorders. *Clinical Psychopharmacology and Neuroscience*. 2015;13(2):188-193.
doi:10.9758/cpn.2015.13.2.188.
https://www.ncbi.nlm.nih.gov/pubmed/26243847

Other Books and Projects

by Tiago Henriques

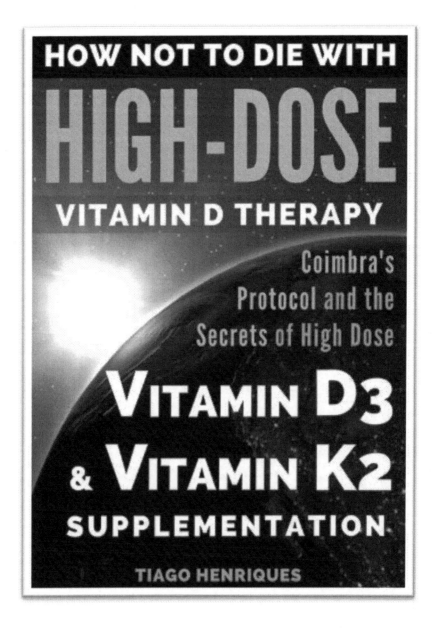

Can Vitamin D kill you?

Did you know the highest Vitamin D recommended daily allowance (RDA) is only **800 IU**?

What if you were told to take **50,000 IU, 100,000 IU** or even **200,000 IU**?

Do you think it would be possible to do this **safely**?

Most Doctors believe vitamin D levels shouldn't be above **100 ng/mL**. What if your blood work said **2000 ng/mL, 3000 ng/mL** or even more? Would you panic?

Welcome to the world of true high-dose vitamin D therapy. A therapy taking the Portuguese speaking world by storm and **helping** people with diseases as serious as multiple sclerosis, rheumatoid arthritis, lupus, among many other autoimmune diseases, with **95%** success.

In addition, the risk of myocardial infarction lowers by **50%** between those subjected to an angiography. The risk of colon cancer can drop up to **80%** and the risk of breast cancer by up to **83%** — imagine! Millions of men and women could still be alive if only they had known about vitamin D in advance. Nevertheless, **more than 1 billion people have insufficient vitamin D levels**. Are you one of them?

What if you knew how to uncover the **exact** dose your body needs and how to supplement this dose safely?

Imagine how things could be different for you.

In this book, we explore in detail the protocols of **Dr. Cícero Coimbra** and physicians like **Dr. Manuel Pinto Coelho**. Names mostly unknown to the English-speaking world **who are revolutionizing medical treatment protocols.**

You will learn everything you need to master, **step-by-step**, in a practical guide written in a clear language. Through many simple illustrations and **easy-to-understand** diagrams you will effortlessly learn:

- How Vitamin D heals.

- The **real dangers** of true high-dose therapy.

- How to **avoid** these dangers.

- What laboratory tests must be done regularly.

- How to interpret the results of these tests and guarantee any side effects are kept at bay while you reap the benefits.

- What supplements to take.

- How each of these supplements relates to vitamin D.

Also, **a simplified version of the protocols** is provided to you. You will know exactly the *why* behind each recommendation. Think about it.

This means there will be no space for analysis-paralysis and that makes all the difference. Moreover, each key statement comes accompanied by references to recent clinical studies from scientifically accredited sources.

Nothing of importance is left unexplained or without a reference.

Seeing how everything fits together in a logical manner, you will be ready to share this life-saving information with others, including your doctor.

You will get clear, scientifically validated, answers to each of the key   questions:

- How can I know **my** body is getting its optimal vitamin D dose?

- How can I keep myself **safe** while taking this dosage?

- How can I be **sure** true high-dose vitamin D therapy actually **works**?

- What is the relationship between vitamin D and vitamin K2?

- How many types of Vitamin K2 there are and how should I supplement them?

All these secrets from the **Portuguese and Brazilian protocols** are finally answered in a simple and direct way in **a single book** in the English-language. A book designed to help you understand everything you need to **know from the very first day.**

This practical guide is built upon **more than 300 references**, providing detailed information on **depression, autism, cancer, osteoporosis, diabetes, autoimmune diseases, fibromyalgia and chronic pain, cardiovascular diseases**, among other health problems.

Unravel the mysteries of vitamin D and vitamin K2 and **reap the benefits of true high-dose therapy while keeping yourself safe.**

Both Kindle and paperback editions are available on Amazon:

- Amazon.com: **www.amazon.com/dp/B07F7LPWML**

- Amazon.co.uk: **www.amazon.co.uk/dp/B07F7LPWML**

Did You Know?

This book was translated and published independently. That means there is no publisher behind. This has its advantages, but one fundamental disadvantage is that there is no national marketing campaign promoting this book.

How can you help?

If you enjoyed this exploration of the secrets of vitamin D and believe in the value of the information provided, what do you think about leaving a review on Amazon? Your words will help others understand the benefits they can reap from the information contained in this book.

On the other hand, if there's any information that you don't agree with or if you need additional information, feel free to contact me at:

- tiagohenriques@academiaciencia.com

Also, if you know about a case study or published clinical trial or another relevant piece of information you'd like to share with me, please do so.

Finally, any tips on how to improve the quality of this translation would be greatly appreciated so feel free to send me your valuable insights.

Contact me using the above email address and I'd be more than happy to read your kind words.

To conclude, I do have a **Portuguese YouTube channel**, https://www.youtube.com/c/CienciaDesenhada, where you can find instructional videos in a whiteboard animation style.

Also, I've published more research and educational material on Udemy and Amazon. However, these are currently available exclusively in Portuguese.

I have plans to eventually translate my works into English and other languages. It'll all be possible thanks to people like you. So, let me show my appreciation for the time you took to analyze this work.

I hope this valuable research can make a real difference in your health and quality of life.

Let me know how it goes for you,

Tiago Henriques

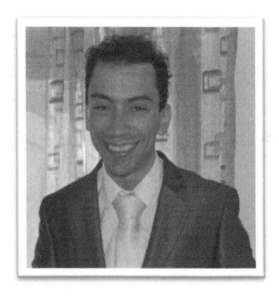

Bibliography

Aston MC. Aspergers in Love, Couple Relationships and Family Affairs. Jessica Kingsley Publishers; 2003.

Attwood T. The Complete Guide to Asperger's Syndrome. Jessica Kingsley Publishers; 2008.

Burns DD. When Panic Attacks, The New, Drug-Free Anxiety Therapy That Can Change Your Life. Harmony Books; 2007.

Ekman P. Emotions Revealed, Second Edition, Recognizing Faces and Feelings to Improve Communication and Emotional Life. Macmillan; 2007.

Goleman D. Emotional Intelligence. Bantam; 2005.

Grandin T. The Way I See it, A Personal Look at Autism & Asperger's. Future Horizons; 2011.

Grandin T, Panek R. The Autistic Brain, Helping Different Kinds of Minds Succeed. 2014.

Grandin T, Attwood T. Different. Not Less, Inspiring Stories of Achievement and Successful Employment from Adults With Autism, Asperger's, and ADHD. Future Horizons; 2012.

Grandin T, Barron S. Unwritten Rules of Social Relationships. 2017

Henriques T. How Not to Die with True High-Dose Vitamin D Therapy, Coimbra's Protocol and the Secrets of Safe High-Dose Vitamin D3 and Vitamin K2 Supplementation. Amazon Digital Services LLC; 2018

Kahneman D. Thinking, Fast and Slow. Macmillan; 2011.

Kaufman RK. Autism Breakthrough, The Groundbreaking Method That Has Helped Families All Over the World. St. Martin's Griffin; 2015.

Kaufman BN. Son-rise, The Miracle Continues. H J Kramer; 1994.

Rosenberg MB. Non Violent Communication. Nonviolent Communication Guide; 2015.

Simone R. Aspergirls, Empowering Females with Asperger Syndrome. Jessica Kingsley Publishers; 2010.

Simone R. 22 Things a Woman with Asperger's Syndrome Wants Her Partner to Know. Jessica Kingsley Publishers; 2012.

Simone R. 22 Things a Woman Must Know If She Loves a Man with Asperger's Syndrome. Jessica Kingsley Publishers; 2009

Simone R, Grandin T. Asperger's on the Job, Must-have Advice for People with Asperger's Or High Functioning Autism, and Their Employers, Educators, and Advocates. Future Horizons; 2010.

Stanford A. Troubleshooting Relationships on the Autism Spectrum, A User's Guide to Resolving Relationship Problems. Jessica Kingsley Publishers; 2013.

35300740R00097

Made in the USA
Middletown, DE
04 February 2019